your guide to
Alzheimer's disease

Extracts in this book have been taken from
*Alzheimer's Disease and Memory Loss Explained:
A Guide for Patient's and Carers* by Alistair Burns,
Sean Page and Jane Winter.
Altman Publishing Ltd, Hertfordshire, 2001.
(ISBN 1860360173)

The ROYAL
SOCIETY *of*
MEDICINE

your guide to
Alzheimer's disease

Professor Alistair Burns

MBChB, FRCP, DHMSA, FRCPsych, MPhil, MD

with

Sean Page and Jane Winter

Hodder Arnold

A MEMBER OF THE HODDER HEADLINE GROUP

Orders: please contact Bookpoint Ltd, 130 Milton Park, Abingdon, Oxon OX14 4SB. Telephone: (44) 01235 827720. Fax: +44 (0) 1235 400454. Lines are open 09.00–17.00, Monday to Saturday, with a 24-hour message answering service. You can also order through our website www.hoddereducation.com

British Library Cataloguing in Publication Data
A catalogue record for this title is available from the British Library.

ISBN-10: 0 340 90501 8
ISBN-13: 9 780340 905012

First published   2005
Impression number   10 9 8 7 6 5 4 3
Year   2008 2007 2006

Copyright © Alistair Burns 2005

Hodder Headline's policy is to use papers that are natural, renewable and recyclable products and made from wood grown in sustainable forests. The logging and manufacturing processes are expected to conform to the environmental regulations of the country of origin.

Every effort has been made to trace copyright for material used in this book. The authors and publishers would be happy to make arrangements with any holder of copyright whom it has not been possible to trace successfully by the time of going to press.

Contents

Acknowledgements

I am most grateful to my close colleagues, Sean Page, Clinical Nurse Specialist in Old Age Psychiatry, and Jane Winter, Senior Clinical Neuropsychologist from the Memory Clinic at Wythenshawe Hospital, without whom this book could not have been prepared. Also to Professor John O'Brien at the University of Newcastle for providing the MRI images, to Catherine Coe and Katie Archer from Hodder, who guided me through the project, to the reviewer who had some excellent suggestions on how the book could be improved and, most of all, to my long-suffering assistant, Barbara Dignan, without whom the project would definitely not have been completed.

Preface

This new book, published in partnership with the Royal Society of Medicine, provides detailed, useful and up-to-date information on Alzheimer's disease. It contains expert yet user-friendly advice, with such useful features as:

Key Terms: demystifying the jargon
Questions and Answers: answering the burning questions
Myths and Facts: debunking the misconceptions
My Experience: how it feels to live with, or care for someone with, this condition.

Bearing the hallmark of excellence and accessibility that characterizes the work of the Royal Society of Medicine, this important guide will enable you and your family to gain some control over the way your Alzheimer's disease is managed by being better informed.

Peter Richardson
Director of Publications, Royal Society of Medicine

Introduction

Alzheimer's disease in the recent past has received unprecedented public attention as a result of high profile individuals suffering from the disease (for example, Ronald Reagan and Iris Murdoch), but also as a result of media attention stemming from the National Institute of Clinical Excellence's draft guidance suggesting that the anti-Alzheimer drugs should not be available on the National Health Service (NHS). With this seepage of information into the public domain, everybody has become more aware of memory problems, their effects on individuals and carers, and their implications in terms of diagnosis, both for themselves and for their relatives.

Because the symptoms of Alzheimer's disease are primarily emotional and behavioural rather than physical, they can be surrounded by an air of mysticism coupled with the fact that probably one of our most basic fears is loss of function and loss of independence, leading to incoherence.

It seemed timely to have a publication dealing specifically with dementia and one of its most common causes, Alzheimer's disease, in particular. Hopefully the information provided here will be of use to people suffering from memory problems, people already diagnosed as having dementia, their families, relatives and carers. I hope the information in this book is of interest and help to anyone reading it.

CHAPTER

1

What is Alzheimer's disease?

Dementia

Alzheimer's disease is a type of **dementia**, and dementia is a medical condition in which there is a serious deterioration in a person's intellectual ability and emotional state. Dementia defines the presence of a particular cluster of symptoms and signs. A symptom is something that a patient complains of, for example, pain or constipation. A sign is something which a doctor notices or uncovers during a clinical examination, for example, raised blood pressure or an abnormal heartbeat. A syndrome is a condition that has a recognizable number of signs and symptoms. Dementia is a syndrome.

dementia
A condition of the brain, with a number of causes, which gives rise to memory loss and emotional changes and results in a person having difficulty looking after themselves.

Symptoms of dementia

These can be described under three headings: loss of memory and higher brain functions; **psychiatric symptoms** and

psychiatric symptoms
Symptoms such as depression, delusions, hallucinations and misidentification seen in people with dementia.

**behavioural
disturbances**
Behaviours such as
wandering, agitation,
aggression and sexual
disinhibition are seen
in people with
dementia.

myth
Everybody, if they lived long
enough, would get
dementia.

fact
Although dementia is a very
common condition (affecting
about 6 per cent of people
over the age of 65), that still
means that 94 per cent do
not have dementia. Even in
people over the age of 90,
where the proportion rises to
as many as one in three or
one in four, studies suggest
that the rate begins to level
off at this age. So, dementia
is not an inevitable
consequence of ageing.

reduplication
When a person
suffering from
Alzheimer's disease
thinks that there are
two of something – an
object or a person –
usually something
which has emotional
significance to the
sufferer.

behavioural disturbances; and activities of
daily living.

Loss of memory and higher brain functions

Loss of memory occurs in all people with
Alzheimer's disease. It is often the first symptom
and gradually gets worse. Often others notice
someone's memory loss before the actual person
does. It may be that someone forgets a
birthday or an anniversary or begins to forget
appointments. Of course, these can be normal
experiences, particularly as people get older, but
if they are severe and, most importantly, if they
get worse over time and more than one would
expect with age-related changes, this suggests
that someone has dementia. People's judgement
can become impaired and they can find it
progressively more difficult to make complex and
important decisions. They can find it increasingly
difficult to handle their own affairs, particularly
financial ones. People can also have problems
understanding language and expressing
themselves, as well as experiencing difficulty in
recognizing other people and, when the
Alzheimer's disease is severe, they need help to
wash, dress and feed themselves.

Q **A few months ago my mother, who has
Alzheimer's disease, began to think that she
had two houses. Why is this?**

A This type of symptom occurs in 10 to 15 per cent of
people with Alzheimer's disease and is based on
damage to that part of the brain which recognizes
things and is called a **reduplication**, i.e. when
people think there are two of things. A house is
probably the most common object of this

A reduplication idea but occasionally it can be with people (usually a spouse) or a pet and is usually something which has emotional significance for the person. What seems to happen is that the part of the brain that is in charge of recognizing things fails and then there is a complex loop of nerve cell activity where the brain tries to make sense of this failure. So, for example, if something in a house does not seem quite right, at a subconscious level the brain thinks there must be two houses — one is completely perfect and the other is slightly different. Because of the dementia and the damage to the brain, the person is unable to integrate and make sense of these two opposing ideas and so the idea is formed that there are two of things. Often the symptoms cause very little distress and it is just something the person says. However, occasionally, it can become very distressing and taking the person for a walk away from the house that is allegedly the wrong one can often alleviate the problem so that, by the time the person returns, the idea seems to have been lost and everything is back to normal.

Psychiatric symptoms and behavioural disturbances

There is a whole host of psychiatric and psychological symptoms and disturbances in behaviour that accompanies Alzheimer's disease. The common ones include:

> **neuropsychiatric symptoms**
> A number of psychiatric or psychological symptoms and behavioural disturbances seen in dementia.

✧ *Depression* – this is very common and about one third of people with Alzheimer's disease have significant **depression**. In addition, it is known that an episode of depression earlier in life is a risk factor for the development of Alzheimer's disease in later life

> **depression**
> A state of lowered mood seen commonly in people with dementia.

✧ *Delusions* – these are fixed ideas, which are usually false but are held intensively and a person with Alzheimer's cannot be dissuaded from them. Common delusions are that people have stolen the sufferer's possessions or that people wish to annoy or harm the sufferer

✧ *Other symptoms* – these include **hallucinations**

✧ *Behavioural disturbances* – there are many types of behavioural disturbance such as aggression (this can be verbal aggression, such as shouting and screaming, or physical aggression such as hitting or punching), agitation (where a person appears very restless and is unable to sit contentedly and at peace) and wandering (a person may walk out of their own home, forget where they are and walk for miles, or if a person is in a nursing or residential home, they may walk around the home constantly).

Activities of daily living

The final expression of Alzheimer's disease is where people are unable to look after themselves and complete, without help, what are called **activities of daily living**. These are things like getting dressed, going to the toilet, brushing one's teeth, combing one's hair and eating a meal. In the early stages of Alzheimer's disease, problems with activities of daily living may be shown by an inability to carry out tasks such as shopping independently, using the telephone, handling money and driving. It is a popular misconception to assume that a person with Alzheimer's disease has simply 'forgotten' how to do these things. The situation is more complex than this and to carry out these tasks the brain needs to do more than simply remember how they were carried out the

hallucinations
Experiences such as visual or auditory hallucinations (seeing or hearing things when there is nothing there) seen in people with dementia.

activities of daily living
Things which we carry out in our everyday lives and which are affected in someone suffering from dementia. Examples include dressing, feeding, washing, eating, handling money, shopping, driving and using the telephone.

last time. The brain needs to be able to co-ordinate all these activities quickly and without interruption and to integrate all the information which is coming in from outside stimuli.

Alzheimer's disease

The two most common causes of dementia are **Alzheimer's disease** and vascular dementia. Alzheimer's disease is caused by the laying down of abnormal proteins in the brain that interfere with its proper functioning by disturbing the way in which the nerve cells communicate with each other. About 60 per cent of people with dementia have Alzheimer's disease.

> **Alzheimer's disease**
> The most common cause of dementia affecting about 60 per cent of people with dementia.

Symptoms of Alzheimer's disease

> **myth**
> People who are very intelligent don't get Alzheimer's disease.

✧ Memory loss, forgetfulness
✧ Impaired judgement
✧ Difficulty in performing tasks, for example, shopping, handling money, using the telephone, working domestic appliances especially if they are new
✧ Problems with language
✧ Disorientation to time and place
✧ Problems with abstract thinking
✧ Changes in mood and behaviour
✧ Changes in personality
✧ Loss of initiative
✧ Depression
✧ Anxiety
✧ Sleep disturbance
✧ Delusions (false ideas, for example, that someone is stealing a person's possessions).

Not everyone with Alzheimer's disease will get all these symptoms and if a person has these

> **fact**
> There is some evidence that high educational achievement can be protective against the development of Alzheimer's disease. The reasons for this are unclear, but it may be something to do with the protective effect of using your brain actively throughout your life. However, dementia can affect people who have achieved very high status and positions – Ronald Reagan, the ex-President of the United States, died in 2004 of Alzheimer's disease, and Bernard Levin, the writer and commentator, also died of the disease in 2004.

symptoms, it does not necessarily mean they have Alzheimer's disease or will get it in the future.

Signs of Alzheimer's disease

The following are things that a doctor will detect on examination:

confusion
A commonly used term indicating, usually, that a person does not know where they are and/or does not know the date, and/or does things which are inappropriate.

✧ Poor results on tests of memory
✧ Disorientation to time and place
✧ Failure to recognize people
✧ **Confusion**
✧ Difficulty with language, such as naming objects
✧ Evidence of depression
✧ Abnormal beliefs.

These changes can be due to a number of different causes and although the end result of these very different processes may be similar, the treatments and the progression of the illness in individual conditions are different. It is therefore very important for a doctor to know the type of dementia from which a person suffers and so tests, examinations and investigations have to be carried out to determine the cause.

Q **I heard once that people who pick their nose are more likely to get Alzheimer's disease. Is this true?**

A There was one case control study a number of years ago that did in fact show such an association. Although is sounds very far fetched, it probably isn't as daft as it seems. The brain is protected by several millimetres of very thick bone. However, at its most vulnerable the space between the outside and the inside of the brain is only a few millimetres thick and is made of thin bone. This area is called the cribriform plate and is at the top of the nose. Although it may sound

A fanciful, some people suggested that infections at the end of a finger could be introduced to the brain through this plate and there was some supporting evidence to suggest that the changes in the brain in Alzheimer's disease started at the front (where the cribriform form plate is) and extended to the back. However, the association has not been confirmed with other studies.

Vascular dementia

Vascular dementia is caused by a hardening of the blood vessels in the brain which results in poor blood flow to the brain and damage (and sometimes death) of some of the brain cells. If an area of brain dies, a stroke occurs. Therefore, this form of dementia can be caused by a stroke. In the 1970s it was considered that to have vascular dementia you needed to suffer one or two big strokes. However, it has become apparent over the last 20 years that people can have vascular dementia without having had strokes and the onset of progression in this situation can be quite slow and insidious, rather like Alzheimer's disease. Even if someone has a stroke, it does not necessarily give rise to any symptoms, and it can often be found as an incidental finding on a brain scan, or even after someone has died, at postmortem. It is important to differentiate people with vascular dementia from people with Alzheimer's disease, because the treatment is very different. There are a few tell-tale signs that people may have vascular dementia. The symptoms may start very quickly and tend to vary from day to day. At times, people will say that a relative appears to be back to normal. There may be a history of a stroke or a transient ischaemic attack (a mini-stroke where the symptoms last

vascular dementia
The second most common cause of dementia affecting about 20 per cent of people with dementia.

myth
It is not possible to have a diagnosis of both Alzheimer's and vascular dementia.

fact
It is increasingly common for people to have features of Alzheimer's and vascular dementia. A brain scan can be helpful at differentiating the two but frequently they occur together.

less then 24 hours). A person may have a history of high blood pressure or heart disease, raised cholesterol, or diabetes. About 20 per cent of people with dementia have vascular dementia. Alzheimer's disease and vascular dementia can exist together in the same person.

Other types of dementia

Lewy body dementia

A type of dementia caused by deposits of protein called Lewy bodies.

frontal lobe dementia

A type of dementia caused by shrinkage in the front part of the brain.

The two less common types of dementia are **Lewy body dementia**, which is caused by an abnormal protein deposit between the nerve cells (similar to but not the same as the protein deposited in Alzheimer's disease) and gives rise to symptoms such as muscle stiffness and tremor as you might see in Parkinson's disease; and **frontal lobe dementia**, which is caused by a specific shrinkage of cells in the front part of the brain and results in change in a person's personality and behaviour.

Q **My mother has Parkinson's disease and memory loss. Could she be developing dementia?**

A It is quite common for people with Parkinson's disease to develop memory problems and loss of concentration. It is important to get a thorough evaluation of your mother's condition to make sure she is not suffering from depression which can cause lapses of concentration and can give symptoms similar to those of dementia. It is also common for people with Parkinson's disease to have symptoms of memory loss due to Parkinson's disease itself. If the symptoms of memory loss are severe and are accompanied by the other symptoms of dementia such as problems with activities of daily living, the development of a dementia is a possibility. There is a particular condition called dementia with Lewy bodies which is associated with features of Parkinson's disease and particular symptoms of dementia such as

> **A** intermittent confusion and visual hallucinations (seeing things when there is nothing there), and paranoid ideas. It is important to recognize this particular type of dementia as treatment can be different from that of uncomplicated Alzheimer's disease or vascular dementia.

Lewy body type dementia

This describes a particular type of dementia, characterized by:

✧ Episodes of delirium (i.e. brief episodes of deterioration in memory)
✧ Falls
✧ Symptoms of Parkinson's disease (when symptoms of Parkinson's disease are present but a person is not considered to have the disease, they are called Parkinsonian symptoms – the most common ones are mild tremor at rest, and stiffness of the muscles)
✧ A number of psychiatric symptoms, such as paranoid ideas (the idea that someone is trying to harm or come after the individual), and visual hallucinations (when someone sees something but there is nobody and nothing there)
✧ An exaggerated reaction to neuroleptic drugs which causes stiffness of the muscles.

Alzheimer's disease is named after the doctor, Alois Alzheimer, who first described it in 1907. He was both a psychiatrist and pathologist and he found deposits of protein between nerve cells in the brain of a person with dementia. Interestingly, when these areas of protein are found in a central region of the brain (called the basal ganglia), the patient will have the symptoms of Parkinson's disease. It is important to make a diagnosis of

Q **Do people suffering from vascular dementia have more insight than people suffering from Alzheimer's disease?**

A It used to be said that because the problems with vascular dementia were more patchy than in Alzheimer's disease, people had more insight into their condition and therefore may be more distressed. Undoubtedly, people with Alzheimer's disease, especially in the early stages, do have insight into their problems, and this is clearly very distressing, not only for them but also for their carers. In the later stages of dementia, insight tends to be lost, and many people say that is a good thing.

Lewy body dementia because some of the drugs which are given to people with dementia to control troublesome symptoms, such as agitation and aggression, can provoke a very severe reaction in people with Lewy body dementia.

Frontal lobe dementia

This is where the front parts of the brain are affected by shrinkage of unknown cause. Symptoms here are slightly different in that changes in personality are very prominent, and sometimes the person can have problems with language. Memory tends not to be affected very early on. People with this disease can behave quite bizarrely at times.

myth
Using aluminium saucepans causes Alzheimer's disease.

fact
Aluminium is a neurotoxin (which means that, given in sufficient quantities, it can damage the nerve cells or neurons). Patients who underwent renal dialysis, when it was first developed, used to get high levels of aluminium in the brain and displayed symptoms of dementia. However, although aluminium can affect the way the brain works, there is no evidence to suggest that it is the cause of Alzheimer's disease. (Someone would have to eat a large number of aluminium saucepans to develop toxic levels of aluminium in the brain!)

How common is dementia?

Dementia affects about 6 per cent of people over the age of 65 but becomes much more common as people get older, affecting as many as one in three or one in four people over the age of 90. In the UK, there are about 800,000 people with dementia of whom just over half have Alzheimer's disease.

Table 1 Causes of dementia

Alzheimer's disease	60%
Vascular dementia	20%
Lewy body dementia	15%
Frontal lobe dementia and other causes	5%

myth
Depression and Alzheimer's disease can't exist together.

fact
It is very common for symptoms of depression to occur in the early stages of Alzheimer's disease, possibly because the person senses their abilities are beginning to fail and they get what is called a reactive depression. Up to two-thirds of people with Alzheimer's disease get depressed at some stage of the illness but these symptoms can be treated effectively and safely with drugs.

my experience

An Alzheimer's disease sufferer

I retired two years ago and was looking forward to spending the time tending my roses in the garden and looking after our grandchildren. It took me quite a few weeks to finally separate myself from work as I always wanted to go in and see how things were going (I don't think I believed they could manage without me). It was after about a year that I noticed that I kept on losing my keys. It wasn't once every couple of weeks which I've always done, it was every second or third day. I'd put them down somewhere and completely forget where they were. There was also an embarrassing incident when my wife and I went to a party and met some new people and I just could not remember their names, even though I tried repeating them when I was introduced. The other frustrating thing is that we had to get a new dishwasher and I can't for the life of me work it. It has lots of different cycles and there are two knobs that you have to get in exactly the right place or it just doesn't work. I've tried reading the instructions but just can't do it. Finally, after several months I was referred to a memory clinic and they told me I had very mild Alzheimer's disease. It's changed my life but at least I know what is wrong and can make some plans for the future as I'm very scared for the day when I won't be able to manage at all.

The wife of the sufferer

My husband retired two years ago and said all he wanted to do was to spend his retirement looking after our grandchildren and pottering about in the garden with his roses. He had only been retired a few months when I began to notice that he kept on asking me for the keys and he seemed to have lost confidence in what he was doing. He withdrew into himself and, once at a party when he couldn't remember someone's name, he got very irritated and said he wasn't going to go to anymore parties ever again, which is a shame because I like going out and now that he's retired we tend to be stuck in together all the time, which I don't think is good for us. We had to get a new dishwasher because he broke the last one and he just cannot get it to work. I don't really want to have to buy a new one and so I found it easier just to say that I would do it. I feel a bit guilty because he's always done the dishes but I can't let him ruin a brand new £300 dishwasher can I? After a while he was referred to a clinic and they said he had Alzheimer's disease. In some ways now he's a lot better because he's accepted the fact that his memory isn't what it should be and he has come to terms with it. He still likes to potter around in the garden but he can't do quite as much as he used to. I'm worried about him driving as well but he became quite irritable the other day when I mentioned that he might have to give that up. I think he may be depressed and when I went to the doctor they put him on an antidepressant but they didn't seem to do him any good and he got an upset stomach.

Are people with Alzheimer's disease living longer?

There is some evidence to suggest that the survival time of people with Alzheimer's disease is greater than it was a few years ago. However, it is quite complicated to interpret the evidence for a number of reasons. There are differences in the way that dementia is diagnosed these days compared to a number of years ago and so it may be that groups of patients are not comparable. The diagnosis of dementia tends to be a bit of a moveable feast with some people being diagnosed relatively early in their illness and some people diagnosed relatively late. Thus, any estimate of survival from time of diagnosis will depend on how long a person has been ill before that diagnosis is made. Sometimes it can be quite difficult to accurately date when the first symptoms began that were attributable to the dementia. Even taking these things into consideration, there is some evidence that patients with dementia are living longer than they did a number of years ago. This is due to improved general medical care and there is also a suggestion that people taking anti-dementia drugs may live longer, possibly as a result of slowing the deterioration of the disease and perhaps by keeping people out of residential and nursing homes.

CHAPTER

2

Memory problems

Noticing changes

If a person notices a change in their memory there are a few important things to think about and consider.

Duration

Any problem with memory needs to be interpreted in the light of its duration. Everybody forgets things from time to time and one or two isolated examples spread over a couple of weeks are probably of little or no significance. Also, a person may be someone who has had a memory problem all their life, and something that has been going on for 30 or 40 years and has not changed is unlikely to be important. It is just a part of the make-up of that person that they need to learn to live with. Most people with Alzheimer's disease describe an onset of memory loss which goes on over a few months. Any problem with memory that has been around for, say, six or nine months and is getting worse should be investigated further.

General health

It is important for the person to consider what their general health is like. It is very common to develop a poor memory if you are physically unwell, especially with a serious disease. Such people can suffer from episodes of confusion that are short-lived periods of disorientation and memory loss that usually disappear when the underlying physical illness is treated. Any severe and disabling illness can give rise to memory loss, however, it is important to remember that if memory loss is severe and deteriorating not to just put it down to the effects of the illness without any further consideration.

Family history

There is some evidence that dementia runs in families. There are two main ways in which this can occur. First, there are a few families where the disease is passed from generation to generation, and second where there is a general increase in the risk of a person developing dementia if there is another member of the family who also has the disease.

From generation to generation

In the first situation, the disease is similar to other inherited characteristics such as brown eyes or blonde hair. There are a few families in the world where large family trees have been built up and the dementia is clearly passed from generation to generation in this way. In this case, the disease usually comes on when people are in their forties and fifties and tends to be a rather severe form of illness. In general, these families account for only about 2 per cent of all cases of Alzheimer's disease. In some cases, it is possible to have a blood test to determine whether you carry the gene to develop Alzheimer's disease.

Q My mother had dementia. Will I get it?

A There is good evidence that dementia does run in families but so do other diseases like stroke, heart disease, asthma and cancer. In some cases, there seems to be a strong genetic predisposition to get dementia but this usually happens when a number of family members are affected and the disease has started at a relatively young age (in people's forties or fifties). Just having one parent who developed dementia when they were quite elderly (in their seventies or eighties), or even an aunt or uncle, probably does not significantly increase a person's risk of getting dementia but if, say, two out of four or three out of six of your mother and your uncles and aunts on your mother's side developed dementia at a relatively young age, it might be worth seeking specialist advice about the situation.

autosomal dominant condition

A condition passed from generation to generation even if only one parent is affected. (An autosomal recessive condition needs both parents to be affected for it to be passed on.)

In these rare situations, one can identify a single genetic mutation on one of the chromosomes which seems to cause Alzheimer's disease. Often, the situation occurs when a number of people in one family are affected by the disease, for example, in an **autosomal dominant condition** 50 per cent of family members can be affected with the disease. So, out of six brothers and sisters, three could have dementia. Where there is a very clear family history of the disease, it can sometimes be helpful to identify specific genetic abnormalities.

The primary purpose of this is to inform people who are young whether they are likely to develop dementia or not as they get older or not and, sometimes, for people to decide whether they should have children. These are obviously very personal decisions and judgements to make and anyone who is considering obtaining these kinds of tests should be referred to an expert genetic counsellor because a great deal of preparation, information and counselling is needed both before and after any tests are done.

Afflicted family member

The second, and by far the most common way in which the disease affects families is that it tends to occur more commonly when there is another family member already affected although, unlike the situation above, it is not possible to be certain. It is comparable to the situation where heart disease, cancer and stroke tends to run in families. There is no blood test in this situation that will be able to tell someone whether or not they will develop Alzheimer's disease.

There is a blood test that tests for apolipoprotein E, which can sometimes be done. This is a protein which everybody has in their blood that helps the blood to carry cholesterol around the body. There are several normal variants which are present in everybody, and possessing one of them is a risk factor for Alzheimer's disease. However, people without this particular genetic type can get Alzheimer's disease, and not everybody with this genetic type gets Alzheimer's disease. It is not a helpful test in the clinical situation when someone is being investigated for the presence of dementia or Alzheimer's disease.

myth
My mother had Alzheimer's disease so I am bound to get it.

fact
While Alzheimer's disease does run in families, it is not passed on from one parent to their children in the general population, although there are some very rare families where it does seem to be inherited like an autosomal dominant condition such as cystic fibrosis.

In practice, one of the more important effects of having a family member who suffers from memory problems, dementia or Alzheimer's disease is that it is likely that another person from that family will come and seek help and treatment far sooner than if there was no family member affected. This is probably because having an affected member of the family will make a person much more aware of the significance and the implication of memory problems, and that is a strong stimulus to seek advice and treatment at an early stage.

Stress

It is common in times of stress to forget one or two things. This is basically because there is too much on a person's mind or there are a few things on that person's mind but they are tending to think about them a lot more than usual. It is important to recognize that stress can cause a variety of symptoms including a temporary loss of memory. Generally, if the memory problem has only been around for a short time, if it is linked clearly in the person's mind to stressful events, or it tends to vary from day to day, or tends to get worse when they are under particular pressure and gets better when they are not under stress, then the memory problem is less sinister and worrisome than it might have been. If at all possible, try to cut down on stress levels. It may be that by becoming aware that stress can cause memory problems, a person might worry less about them and improve in that way!

Depression

It is very common for people suffering from depression to complain of memory problems. However, depression is very much more common in people who have dementia and Alzheimer's disease than in the normal population. If a person has had a previous episode of depression, whether it has been treated by a general practitioner or a specialist, or if they are prone to depression, there should be an awareness that these symptoms may at least contribute to the loss of memory. Some symptoms of depression include: fatigue and tiredness; subjective feelings of the blues; poor appetite; sleep disturbance (particularly waking early in the morning); weight loss (or more rarely, weight gain); loss of enjoyment; not looking forward to things; not enjoying grandchildren; poor concentration; irritability (often noticed by others); feeling worse in the morning; feelings of guilt; or a feeling you have let people down.

If after having considered all these things a person is still worried about their memory problem, the advice must be to go and see a general practitioner (GP). Be prepared to give him or her as much information as possible about current symptoms and past history. Be prepared to have a brief test of memory in the surgery. It is quite in order to take a friend or relative – it is always helpful to have someone else there in case there are things the doctor says which may be forgotten. Write any questions down on a piece of paper to take along.

What happens at your GP's surgery?

A person's GP is the most important person involved with their care. He or she usually knows the patient and their family well and will be the first person the patient sees. They may carry out some investigations such as blood tests. They will be responsible for referring the person for specialist advice and investigations and will monitor the illness and treat any additional symptoms as they emerge.

What happens at a memory clinic?

Memory clinics are now quite common in the UK and are specialist centres attached to hospitals. They will carry out extensive tests and investigations to discover the cause of memory problems and have more access to these tests (such as brain scans) than a GP. Because they see people with memory problems all the time, they will have more experience in this area than the average GP. It is likely that the patient would be seen more than once at a clinic and that they would see different professionals such as nurses, a psychologist, perhaps a social worker and a doctor.

memory clinic
An out-patient clinic specializing in the diagnosis and treatment of people with memory disorders.

If someone has a relative who has memory problems, they may have to take the initiative and persuade the relative to go to get help. The relative may not recognize there is a problem and even if they do, they may not want to acknowledge that they need help. Denying there is anything wrong can sometimes be a very effective defence. Gentle continued pressure is probably the best way of trying to persuade someone to seek help.

my experience

I noticed that my mother's memory had been getting worse for about two years. I am particularly sensitive because my nanna was in her seventies when she developed memory loss. After some persuasion I managed to get my mum to come with me to the doctor.

When we went in, the doctor put my mum at ease immediately and asked her how she was. After a few minutes she asked my mum about her memory and mum admitted that perhaps it wasn't quite what it should be. She asked my mum a few questions about the day and the date, which mum only got partly right but the doctor didn't correct her, which I thought was a good thing, but then when my mum asked whether she had got the answer correct, the doctor was quite honest with her. She asked my mum some questions about what her mood was like and how her physical health was. She asked if mum would mind if someone who specialized in memory problems came to see her at home. To my amazement she said that she would quite like to see someone! The doctor said she would organize some blood tests and that someone would visit sometime over the next two or three weeks.

CHAPTER

3

Identifying dementia and Alzheimer's disease

Diagnosis and assessment

When a person goes to their GP with symptoms of memory loss or other features of dementia, the doctor embarks on a two-stage process. First, the doctor will establish if the person suffers from a dementia and, if that is the case, what is the cause of the dementia. There are a number of different conditions which may mimic the symptoms of dementia and the range of possibilities is called the **differential diagnosis**. Second, is to establish what is the cause of the dementia. Each stage involves taking a careful history by listening to the patient and their family and carers, carrying out a physical and mental state examination and organizing a series of tests and investigations. In practice, the two processes take place at the same time, i.e. the questions and examinations which help the

differential diagnosis
The range of possible conditions that can mimic the symptoms of dementia.

doctor decide whether a person is demented or not can help determine the cause of the dementia.

Differential diagnosis of dementia

The following points need to be taken into consideration when assessing dementia:

✧ Depression
✧ Normal ageing
✧ Mild cognitive impairment
✧ Delirium
✧ Drugs.

Added to this, learning disability (mental handicap), the effects of a poor environment and poor vision and hearing can all make differential diagnosis difficult.

Depression

Depression is a common illness and affects many elderly people. There are two types which are described. The first is severe and usually needs treatment from a doctor or psychologist – it is often referred to as a 'clinical depression'. The proportion of people with clinical depression is about 3 or 4 per cent (i.e. of a survey of 100 people, three or four would have clinical depression), although the proportion might be higher in people, say, who are in hospital or who are in nursing homes. Clinical depression is more severe than minor depression, which is milder and affects up to 20 per cent of people. The symptoms of this type of depression, are relatively minor; they do not last very long and do not cause as much distress or concern to people. It usually does not need to be treated and is self-limiting, although some people's symptoms may progress to become clinical depression. Some of the symptoms of depression are similar to those of people with dementia. People who are depressed often complain of a poor memory, say they lack concentration and are unable to remember things. These symptoms also occur in people with dementia. To make things more complicated, depression can occur in people suffering from dementia. Some people say that this is a natural reaction when a person begins to realize that their memory is failing. When someone goes to their doctor with signs and symptoms of dementia, a careful examination of their mental state is needed to decide whether they are depressed or not. If there is any doubt, most doctors would err on the side of caution and give people a course of antidepressants (a so-called 'treatment trial') and assess whether they get better or not.

Normal ageing

We all know that our memory deteriorates as we get older – many people regard this as an inevitable (and unenviable) result of ageing. When someone is noticed to have a memory problem, the decision has to be made as to whether the person has an illness or not. This sounds obvious, but if the symptoms are very mild and not affecting the way the person is functioning, then there may be no reason to suppose they have an illness. However, if they come along and ask for help it suggests that they are bothered by it.

The way in which dementia is tested is to carry out tests of **cognitive function** (a test of memory and other things like language). If a representative group of people carries out a memory test, one gets what is called 'a normal distribution' of scores. In that way, it is like height and weight – some people have scores at either end, some low and some high, but the vast majority of people score in the middle. This has led some people to say that dementia is not really an illness, it just represents one end of a spectrum. It is not like cancer which someone either does or does not have. Things are not as clear cut in relation to dementia, but there is no doubt that it is possible to identify a group of people who score very badly on tests of cognitive function, who are bothered by it and who have an illness. Also, tests of cognitive function are only one part of how dementia is expressed – there are other aspects of the disorder (problems with activities of daily living, poor judgement and psychiatric symptoms), which are needed to make a diagnosis of dementia and these do not normally occur in the absence of disease.

> **cognitive function**
> Tests of memory, language and mental agility carried out to test the brain's function.

Mild cognitive impairment

This refers to the situation where someone has complaints of memory loss but there is no evidence of dementia. The criteria by which the condition is diagnosed are as follows:

✧ Complaints of memory loss, corroborated by someone who knows the person well

✧ Objective evidence of deficits on neuropsychological tests (i.e. on objective tests of memory, the person scores less than would be expected for someone of that age and sex)

✧ No evidence of dementia (in other words the deficits are not as severe as to affect someone's life in a significant way)

✧ Normal cognitive function other than loss of memory (in other words, the person is still able to manage their affairs completely satisfactorily and their judgement and personality are normal)

✧ No problems with activities of daily living – the person is still able to manage independently and needs no help with things like driving, handling money, organizing business affairs, etc.

Obviously, the doctor has to make sure that there is no emotional cause for the symptoms of memory loss (such as depression) or physical cause that might contribute to them.

The main thing about mild cognitive impairment is that, although the person is not suffering from dementia, they will have a 12–15 times increased chance of developing Alzheimer's disease every year. This has led a lot of people to claim that mild cognitive impairment is in fact the very early stage of Alzheimer's disease and everyone should get treated. It is a little like having slightly raised blood pressure, raised cholesterol, or raised blood sugar, which is not normal but does not merit treatment. One might ask reasonably, why not treat everybody anyway, but any treatment has a risk and it would be inappropriate to treat people for something when there is no evidence that it is effective.

The most important thing is that if someone has a diagnosis of mild cognitive impairment, other conditions should be excluded by the same sorts of tests and investigations described for the investigation of someone with suspected dementia (see page 36). The memory of a person with mild cognitive impairment should also be monitored.

Delirium (an acute confusional state)

In older people, **delirium** is caused by a physical illness and this seems to produce a chemical imbalance in the brain which gives rise to symptoms of confusion. The person has trouble thinking and can appear disorientated (i.e. they do not know where they are and do not know the date, month, year or season). The best way of discriminating delirium from dementia is to enquire how the illness started and how it progressed. In dementia, the illness tends to start slowly and progress slowly, whereas in delirium it starts quickly and the symptoms tend to fluctuate from day to day. Also, in delirium there is almost always a physical cause for the symptoms (i.e. an infection in the chest or in the urine, heart failure or cancer are common causes of delirium). The situation is complicated by the fact that if people who have dementia become physically ill, they are more prone to getting an episode of delirium in addition to their dementia.

Drugs

All drugs have unwanted side effects – symptoms may mimic dementia. People with dementia are probably more prone to suffer from a physical illness and are, generally speaking, more likely to get side effects from

delirium
The acute upset in mental function causing disorientation, confusion and psychiatric symptoms such as auditory and visual hallucination and paranoid ideas. It tends to come on quickly as it is invariably caused by physical illness.

medication. This is especially true if a person is taking more than one drug. A doctor will always consider carefully the drugs a person is taking. If going to see a doctor, always take a list of drugs being taken. Sometimes, stopping a drug for a short time can be helpful in deciding whether it is contributing to, or may be causing, symptoms related to dementia.

Things which make the differential diagnosis difficult

Learning disability (mental handicap)

Dementia is something that people may develop at some point during their life, that is, it is not something a person is born with. People suffering from learning disability have often had their condition since birth and it has led to a lifelong impairment in cognitive functioning. It can be very difficult to assess if a person with learning disability has developed a dementia as the diagnosis rests on demonstrating a change in cognitive function. People with learning disability (particularly **Down's syndrome**) can develop dementia later in life, and often the manifestations of that dementia are more apparent in terms of abnormal behaviour rather than symptoms or complaints of memory loss. There is a specific association between Down's syndrome and Alzheimer's disease in that the majority of patients with Down's syndrome, over the age of 40, develop structural changes in their brains similar to those seen in Alzheimer's disease sufferers.

Down's syndrome

Down's syndrome refers to a congenital disorder where a characteristically flattened facial appearance, short stature and low IQ is present. It is caused by an individual having 3 copies (instead of the normal 2) of chromosome 21. It used to be called Mongolism but this term was regarded as offensive and is now no longer used.

The effects of poor environmental stimulation

Because many of the tests which are used to assess dementia need the person to have a certain degree of initiative, education and general intelligence, occasionally people who have lived in a very unstimulating environment for many years will perform poorly on the tests and may give the impression that they have dementia. These situations are rare. One example would be people who, for some reason, have lived in a long-stay hospital for a long time without much contact with the outside world and not much stimulation. These individuals can appear to have dementia, so the environment in which a person lives must be taken into account when carrying out an assessment.

Poor vision and hearing

It is important to make sure that a person can hear and see as well as they can before they undergo clinical tests. When going for an examination, a person must make sure they take their glasses and hearing aid with them. It is also a good idea to get new batteries for a hearing aid.

Causes of the dementia

It is important that the diagnosis of Alzheimer's disease is communicated sensitively and effectively to the patient and their carers. In some areas, post-diagnostic groups can be an effective way of discussing the many implications that a diagnosis of dementia has for the person themselves and their carers. Once the diagnosis of dementia has been made, the next stage is to assess the cause of the dementia. A logical series of tests and examinations is carried out to exclude illnesses in the rest of the body, some of which are treatable, and to rule out some brain conditions. When this has been done, one decides whether the cause is Alzheimer's disease (60 per cent), vascular dementia (20 per cent) (or a combination of the two), Lewy body dementia (15 per cent) frontal lobe dementia (5 per cent).

Illnesses in the rest of the body

There are a number of different illnesses which appear to affect the brain in ways that can cause symptoms similar to dementia. People who have an underactive thyroid gland can have problems with poor concentration and poor memory. Often there are other signs of an underactive thyroid, such as tiredness, dislike of cold weather, weight gain or thinning of the hair. It can be detected by a simple blood test and replacement treatment with the hormone is easily given in the form of a tablet.

People who have particular deficiencies of certain vitamins can also have symptoms of a dementia. Too little vitamin B12 and folic acid (found in vegetables) can give rise to symptoms of dementia, particularly if the deficiencies are very severe. These deficiencies can sometimes arise because of a bad diet. It is further complicated because some people who have dementia from other causes can neglect their diet and not get enough of these vitamins. Treatment is in the form of tablets for folic acid and injections for vitamin B12. Any general physical illness can give rise to symptoms of dementia, which is why a person with suspected dementia will have a general physical examination and blood test to make sure that medical conditions such as anaemia, liver and kidney problems, diabetes and raised cholesterol in the blood are detected and treated.

Q My doctor said I was deficient in vitamin B12, and that this might contribute to my memory loss. He suggested that I needed injections. Could this be right?

A As part of the blood tests for people being investigated for Alzheimer's disease, two of the common B vitamins in the body are measured – vitamin B12 and folic acid. There is some evidence that low levels of vitamin B12 can affect the memory in that they influence the way that brain cells communicate with each other and can give rise to symptoms of memory loss. However, people who have Alzheimer's disease can be low in vitamin B12 for a number of reasons (such as poor diet or a problem with absorbing food). In this situation, it is always best to increase the level to its optimum to make sure that any symptoms that could be related to B12 deficiency are treated. B12 is a safe drug and you can't overdose on it. It can be given by injection or tablet although it is not absorbed by the stomach very efficiently and injections are the best way to ensure there is a rapid rise in the level of the vitamin in the body. B vitamins are found in fresh vegetables.

Changes within the brain

People may develop brain tumours which can give rise to symptoms of dementia. The symptoms of a brain tumour are often physical, for example, headache or a feeling of sickness, particularly in the morning. They may well have physical symptoms such as loss of muscle power, or tingling in an arm or leg. There are several types of brain tumours, some arising in the brain itself, and others where the tumour has started somewhere else in the body and smaller parts have spread to the brain. Bleeding may occur in the outer covers of the brain, especially after a head injury (bleeding inside the brain gives a stroke).

Brain tumours and bleeding can be detected on a brain scan (see Plate 4) and can sometimes give rise to symptoms suggestive of dementia. If someone has had a severe head injury and the clinical symptoms have come on quite suddenly afterwards, one might suspect that a bleed in the brain has taken place. Repeated head injuries give rise to a form of dementia, found in boxers, called 'dementia pugilistica' (Mohammed Ali suffers from this condition). The other main type of problem which can occur in the brain is called **hydrocephalus** (literally, water on the brain). What happens is that the fluid which bathes the brain inside the skull (the cerebrospinal fluid) flows inside the brain and then through a narrow channel to the outside surface of the brain and down the spinal cord, where it is absorbed into the bloodstream. This fluid is very important in protecting the brain against injury. When there is a blockage to the flow of the fluid from the inside of the brain to the outside, the pressure builds up inside, and the areas inside the brain are forced outwards and upwards by the pressure of fluid. This can occur in some people after a very severe infection of the brain or a type of bleed in the brain which takes place in the outer surface, called a 'subarachnoid haemorrhage'.

In children, because the skull bones have not fused together, there is space with this increasing pressure for the head to get bigger. However, very early on in life the skull binds together and the

hydrocephalus
This refers to an increased amount of the normal fluid (cerebrospinal fluid) which lies around the brain, inside the skull.

increase in pressure merely squashes the brain. It is an important condition to identify, because it can be treated by inserting a tube inside the brain to relieve the pressure. In addition to symptoms of dementia, people with this type of hydrocephalus are often incontinent of urine and are unable to walk very well. For some reason, as the brain shrinks the pressure which is needed to keep the brain enlarged returns to normal, and so the pressure on the inside of the brain is similar to that seen in normal people, hence the name 'normal pressure hydrocephalus' (see Plate 5).

Signs of Alzheimer's disease

As we have seen, this is the most common cause of dementia and affects about 60 per cent of people who suffer from dementia.

It is called Alzheimer's disease after the doctor Alois Alzheimer who described the case of a woman who died when she was aged 51 and had all the symptoms of dementia. She had a post-mortem and, when her brain was examined under the microscope, Alzheimer found two abnormalities: layers of protein in between the nerve cells, and areas of damaged nerve fibres which, instead of being straight, had become tangled. He described the case in a medical journal and, in 1910, his teacher (a psychiatrist called Emil Kraepelin) wrote a book and named the disease after his pupil, Alzheimer. This has led people to imagine that Alzheimer's disease can only be diagnosed after death at a post-mortem.

What happens in reality is that a number of studies have shown associations between the clinical features people have when they are alive and the post-mortem findings after death. These have been put together in the form of 'diagnostic criteria'. Thus, if a person has a particular set of signs and symptoms, as have been highlighted in Chapter 1, pages 5–6, one can be almost certain that they will turn out to have Alzheimer's disease.

Medical diagnosis, like most other things, is not 100 per cent accurate. In practice, what happens is that the doctor will carry out a number of tests to exclude other causes of dementia and, when they have been excluded, he or she can be almost certain that a person does have Alzheimer's disease. The symptoms of Alzheimer's disease characteristically start off gradually and progress gradually. Often when someone comes to the attention of a doctor, they may have had their symptoms for many years. It is often difficult to give an accurate date when the symptoms started.

Q Is there any association between epilepsy and dementia?

A No there is no specific association but epileptic fits get more common in people with dementia as the dementia increases in severity. Fits are treated in the same way as any other fit and this is usually successful. Rarely, some of the anti-dementia drugs may cause fits and this can sometimes happen in a person who has a predisposition towards epilepsy (they may have had a single fit many years earlier but none since).

Possible signs of dementia

Look at the points below to discover if the symptoms experienced suggest Alzheimer's disease.

Do you have problems with any of these activities?

Memory problems

- ✧ Do you forget people's names?
- ✧ Do you forget appointments?
- ✧ Do you forget conversations you have had with people?
- ✧ Do you forget where you have put things?
- ✧ Do you tend to repeat yourself?
- ✧ Do you have trouble paying attention?

(Note – It is very common, particularly as we get older, to have lapses of memory. Remember – if you forget somebody's name, it doesn't mean you have Alzheimer's disease.)

Handling complex tasks

- ✧ Do you have difficulty cooking a meal or organizing for your bills to be paid?
- ✧ Do you have trouble working new pieces of equipment which you or your family have bought?
- ✧ Do you have more trouble adding things up in your head than you used to?
- ✧ Does the crossword take longer to do than it used to?

Reasoning ability

- ✧ Do you tend to get flustered in new situations?
- ✧ Do you have difficulty in solving everyday problems which you used to do without a second thought? For example, would you know what to do if the lights in the house fused?

Disorientation

✧ Do you ever get lost on what are familiar routes?

✧ Do you ever get lost when you are driving?

✧ Have you ever forgotten what day it is and have had to ask somebody?

Behaviour

✧ Have you found yourself more irritable than usual?

✧ Have people commented that your personality seems to have changed?

✧ Do you find yourself less easy-going than you used to be?

Investigations and tests

A fairly set routine is followed when someone suspected of having Alzheimer's disease goes to see their GP or a specialist clinic. Contrary to popular belief and expectation, a diagnosis of dementia and its causes is relatively straightforward. Many people have great faith in expensive brain scans but for the vast majority of people this is neither desirable nor necessary. Of course, there are situations where the diagnosis is particularly difficult or complex and further investigations are needed but, generally, they are not. The main points of the history and examination are outlined below.

History of the illness

The most important first step for a doctor is to take a clinical history from the patient. Patients are usually able to describe their own symptoms, how they started and how they have developed, but if someone has a significant degree of

FRONT

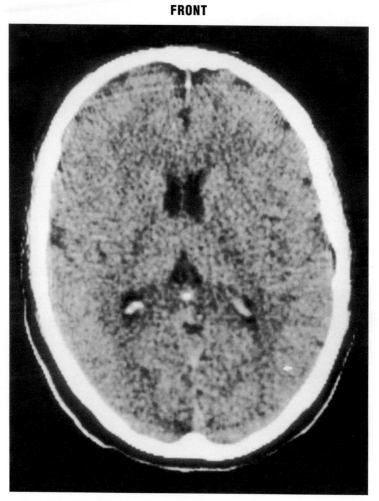

BACK

Plate 1
A CT scan of a normal brain.

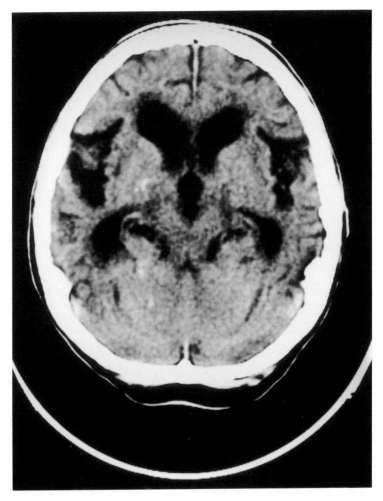

Plate 2

A CT scan showing shrinkage of the brain (atrophy) in Alzheimer's disease.

Areas of black have increased and the grey area of the brain does not extend right up to the white rim of the skull as in Plate 1.

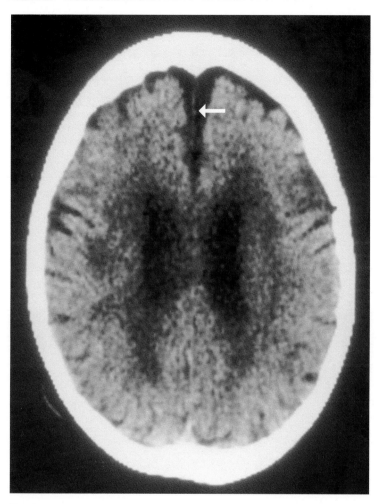

Plate 3
A CT scan showing shrinkage of the front part of the brain.

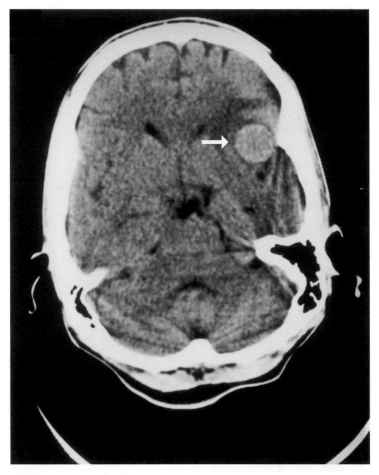

Plate 4
A CT scan showing a brain tumour.

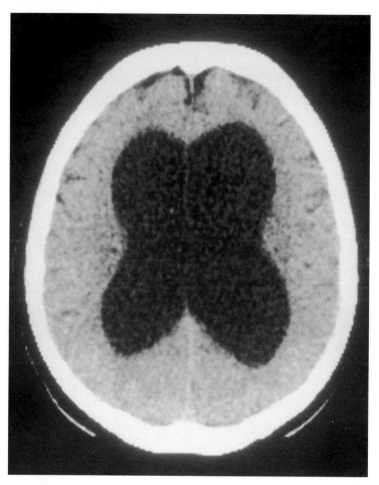

Plate 5
A CT scan showing normal pressure hydrocephalus.

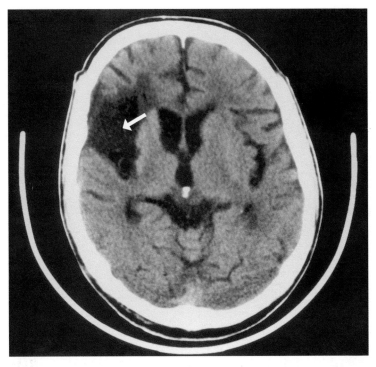

Plate 6
A CT scan showing an area where the brain has died as a result of a cerebral infarction (stroke).

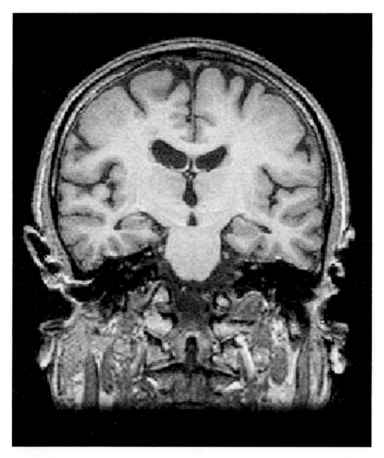

Plate 7
An MRI scan showing a normal brain.
(Courtesy of Professor John O'Brien)

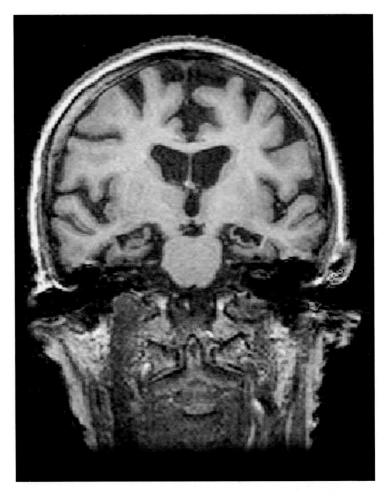

Plate 8
An MRI scan showing atrophy in Alzheimer's disease.
Grey areas of the brain have been replaced and areas of black have increased.
(Courtesy of Professor John O'Brien)

memory loss, disorientation, confusion or dementia, it will be necessary to take the history almost entirely from a relative or carer. Even if the patient is able to describe his or her symptoms accurately, it is always important to check the history out with someone else. The types of question that are asked include:

When did the symptoms start?
What was the first symptom?
Did it start suddenly or gradually?
Has it progressed suddenly or gradually?
Were there any special circumstances around the time the symptoms started?
Is there anything that has made them worse or better?
What is the person's reaction to the symptoms?
Have other people outside the family noticed anything?

A doctor or nurse will often ask some specific questions about particular symptoms from which a patient with dementia might suffer. These would include specific symptoms about depression. For example:

Have you been feeling very tired recently?
Do you find your concentration is poor?
Do you look forward to the future?
Do you feel guilty about anything?
Do you enjoy things?
Do you sleep well at night?
Have you lost weight?
Is there any change in your mood during the day (for example, feeling worse in the morning)?
Have other people said you have been more irritable recently?

delusions
False ideas which are fixed and unshakeable and often seen in people with dementia.

It might be appropriate for the doctor or nurse to ask the patient specific questions about **delusions** and other psychiatric symptoms. It is also important for them to get an idea of what the person can and cannot do in terms of activities of daily living, for example: can they still do the shopping on their own; are they able to handle money; can they still drive safely; are they still as neat and tidy as they used to be; do they comb their hair as much as they used to; or do they need to be reminded to change their clothes?

Examination of the mental state

psychotic symptoms
Symptoms such as delusions, hallucinations and misidentifications.

This consists of questions concerning how a person is feeling and checks out whether an individual is depressed or has any **psychotic symptoms** (ideas or experiences) such as delusions, hallucinations or **misidentifications**. If a person complains of a physical illness then it is necessary to ask some specific questions about physical symptoms.

misidentifications
When a person with dementia does not recognize a person or an object.

When someone is suspected of having dementia, the most important part of the examination is a test of memory. There are a number of standardized tests which are available, or the doctor or nurse might just ask some general questions without recording them in a formal way. Generally, people favour recording memory problems in a formal way.

Whether a scale is used or not, there are a number of questions which are usually asked. These include questions and tests about:

Orientation to time and place

The person is asked to say the date (the day of the week, the month, the year, the season and the date in the month) and also where the person is (does the person know what city or town they are in, do they know their address at home, do they know the district they are in or do they know the name of the hospital they are in?).

> **Q** My husband has Alzheimer's disease and can remember what happened on our wedding day 50 years ago but not what he had for lunch an hour ago. Does this mean he's putting it on?
>
> **A** No, it is very common for things to be remembered that occurred many years ago but not more recent things. It seems that they experience the 'last in, first out' rule.

Memory

Generally this consists of asking a person to repeat three words straight after the interviewer and then the person is asked them again a minute or two later. This tests both immediate memory (registration of memory) and long-term memory (after one or two minutes). This specific test of memory does not relate to what people generally regard as short- and long-term memory (i.e. remembering things that have happened in the past day or the past week is short-term memory and things that happened 30 or 40 years ago is long-term memory). Examples of words used in the test include 'ball', 'car', 'man', 'apple', 'table' and 'penny'.

Concentration

This test can take two forms. Often someone is asked to spell a word backwards, after spelling it forwards. Alternatively, someone is asked to take 7 away from 100 and then carry on decreasing the answer by seven, telling the interviewer each number they get (i.e. the person would say, 93,

86, 79, 72, 65 whereupon the person is generally stopped at this point). If a person has always had difficulty with arithmetic, then counting from 20 down to 1 or saying the months of the year backwards is an alternative. It is often also important to see if the person can tell the interviewer anything that is happening in the news.

Language function

This is tested by asking a person to name a common object, such as a watch, a pen, a tie or a pair of shoes.

Copying

There is often a test to measure if a person can copy a figure. This can be a simple figure such as a triangle or a more complex one such as two intersecting five-sided figures.

Following instructions

The person may be asked to carry out a simple command such as to take a piece of paper in their right hand, fold it in half and put it on the floor.

Clock drawing test

A test which is becoming more popular is to ask a person to draw a clock, which can take a number of different forms. For example, a person is asked to draw a clock face which includes drawing a circle and putting the numbers in, and then putting the hands to show a time, such as ten past ten. This test shows how a particular part of the brain is working.

Mini Mental State Examination

This is probably one of the most popular tests used and gives a score out of 30. It takes about ten minutes to complete.

In specialist settings, more detailed neuropsychological tests are carried out. These can only be given by specialist trained psychology staff and can take anything up to an hour. They provide a very thorough picture of how the brain is functioning.

Physical examination

This takes the form of a general physical examination, which would include checking the pulse and blood pressure, listening to the heart and lungs and testing the reflexes to see if there are any signs of a stroke. In practice, this means tapping on the elbows, wrists, ankle and knees with a tendon hammer. A key is often drawn along the base of the foot to see in which direction the big toe moves (if it moves down it is normal, if it moves up it suggests a person may have had a stroke). The strength of muscles in the arms and legs is also tested and a weakness may indicate that there has been a stroke. A test of co-ordination, such as asking a person to touch their own nose with their index finger and then touch the examiner's finger and then do it repeatedly, may be carried out.

Physical investigations

These usually include a blood test that is subjected to a routine analysis which includes a full blood count (to check there is no anaemia), tests of liver function and kidney function, blood glucose (to test for diabetes), tests of level of thyroid hormone

electrocardiogram (ECG)

A tracing of the heart showing the rate (number of beats per minute) as well as showing if the electrical conduction of the heart is normal. It can also be used to diagnose heart attacks.

electroencephalogram (EEG)

A tracing of the brain waves which can be used to diagnose epilepsy. It can also show where there is shrinkage of the brain and is used to diagnose Creutzfeldt–Jakob disease.

CT scan

A type of brain scan which shows the structure of the brain.

in the blood and vitamin levels (vitamin B12 and folic acid) as well as checking cholesterol levels. A urine sample is often taken to test for evidence of any sugar in the urine or any infections.

A chest X-ray is carried out if the person has symptoms of chest disease and a tracing of the heart (**electrocardiogram, ECG**) is completed if the person has heart symptoms. A tracing of the brain waves (**electroencephalogram, EEG**) is useful as it gives information about the function of the brain's activity. It can show if a person is likely to have a delirium or if they have had a stroke. (Plate 6 shows a scan of a patient's brain who has had a stroke.)

Usually, if someone is suspected of having dementia, a brain scan is carried out. There are two common types of brain scan. A Computed Tomography (or Computed Axial Tomography) scan is the most common. This is known as a **CT** or **CAT scan** and is a non-invasive procedure that can be carried out in about five or ten minutes. It involves lying on a moveable bed and putting your head in what looks like a large washing machine or dishwasher (see Figure 1). Modern scanners tend not to be as enclosed or as claustrophobic as older scanners. Occasionally, there may be a need for an injection which can highlight areas of the brain. The main reason for carrying out a CT or CAT scan is that it can show the structure of the brain and if there is a tumour, clot or haemorrhage. If there is shrinkage of the brain, this can be seen as well and it is sometimes helpful to know if one part of the brain is more shrunken than another part. Compare Plate 1 and Plate 2. Plate 1 shows a perfectly normal healthy brain while Plate 2 shows one with Alzheimer's disease.

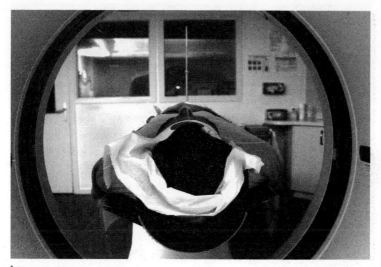

Figure 1 CT scan machine.
(Science Photo Library/AJ Photo/Hop American)

A second type of brain scan is called an **MRI** or **magnetic resonance imaging scan** and uses a slightly different technique from the CT scan. Compare Plates 7 and 8 which show MRI scans of a perfectly normal brain and one with Alzheimer's disease. Because the head is put in a magnet, there are some situations where someone could not have an MRI scan, say, if they have had a previous operation in their brain and a metal clip has been placed on an artery, or if they have a cardiac pacemaker. Also, the apparatus for an MRI scan is much more confining and anyone who suffers from claustrophobia might become anxious or nervous (see Figure 2).

> **MRI scan**
> A type of brain scan which shows the structure of the brain in finer detail compared to a CT scan.

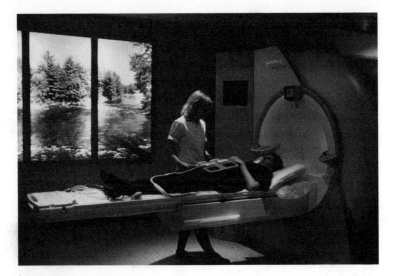

Figure 2 MRI scan machine.
(Science Photo Library/John Cole)

SPET scan
A type of brain scan that shows the blood flow in the brain.

Another type of scan which is sometimes carried out is called a **SPET scan**. SPET stands for Single Photon Emission Tomography (SPECT, for Single Photon Emission Computed Tomography, is the same thing). This is a type of brain scan that shows the blood flow in the brain and contrasts to a CT or MRI scan which show solely the structure of the brain. In SPET, a radioisotope is injected into a vein in the arm and a camera (similar to that used in a CT scan) can give an accurate picture of the level of blood flow to various parts of the brain. It is like looking inside the bonnet of a car – a CT scan or MRI scan is like looking at the engine when it is switched off and a SPET scan is like looking at it with the engine switched on when you can see some bits of the engine moving. A SPET scan is particularly good at showing differences in the blood supply in different parts of the brain, for example, in people with frontal lobe dementia, there is often very little or no blood flow going to the frontal lobes whereas in Alzheimer's disease, blood flow is decreased to the back parts of the brain.

Q **Can a brain scan diagnose Alzheimer's disease?**

A No, but there are a number of types of brain scans, including a computed tomography (CT) scan and a magnetic resonance imaging (MRI) scan. These are helpful in detecting whether there is a brain tumour or stroke, or if there is shrinkage of the brain (as you would see in Alzheimer's disease). However, you cannot diagnose Alzheimer's disease using a scan on its own.

Another type of brain scan which is not used in clinical practice but that you may have heard about is called a PET (positron emission tomography) and this shows the metabolism of the brain.

myth
There is a specific blood test for Alzheimer's disease.

fact
Unfortunately there is no blood test that will diagnose Alzheimer's disease. As part of the assessment of someone with dementia, blood tests are taken. These are to test for diseases which could mimic the symptoms of Alzheimer's disease and also to make sure that a person is generally healthy. A full blood count will see if there are any infections or if the person is anaemic, a measure of the levels of Vitamin B12 and folate will see if there is a vitamin deficiency, a glucose measurement will test for the presence of diabetes, a cholesterol test will be able to tell whether there is any need for treatment to lower cholesterol and, finally, tests for the functioning of the liver and kidneys are usually carried out. In very rare situations where Alzheimer's disease is a genetic condition and is clearly passed from one generation to the next, there are some blood tests that can assess the presence of particular genes which appear, in some cases, to be the cause of Alzheimer's disease. However, these are not used routinely, are not available routinely, and are only given in the setting of very specialist genetic advice and genetic counselling where Alzheimer's disease runs very closely in families.

cerebrospinal fluid

Cerebrospinal fluid is the fluid which bathes the brain – it is inside the brain substance and also around the outside of the brain. It is a way of cushioning the brain from forces from outside. The fluid is manufactured inside the brain and circulates to the outside (still inside the skull) where it is absorbed into the bloodstream. If there is any blockage to that circulation, the amount of fluid under pressure can build up, giving hydrocephalus. In children, before the skull bones have knitted together, this causes an increase in the size of the head but after about 18 months or 2 years of age, the skull is firm and the pressure, as it increases inside, squashes the brain rather than causing the head to enlarge.

Very occasionally, it is necessary to do a lumbar puncture to examine the **cerebrospinal fluid**. This involves a person lying on their side in a bed and having a needle inserted in the base of their spine to draw off some fluid. This is a very safe and routine procedure, although the person usually needs to stay in hospital during the day for this to be carried out.

When a doctor or nurse has all the information available, a 'formulation' is made of an individual case and a diagnosis and treatment plan can be offered.

The difference between vascular dementia and Alzheimer's disease

The difference between vascular dementia and Alzheimer's disease is not a straightforward one. First, the history can be helpful in distinguishing the two. In people with vascular dementia, the onset can be quite sudden with a step-wise decline over time, indicating sudden periods of deterioration, probably equating with episodes of stroke or transient ischaemic attack (where someone gets the symptoms of a stroke such as a paralysis down one side of the body or problems with language but completely recovers within 24 hours) with times of stability. In Alzheimer's disease the decline is consistent and gradual. In vascular dementia there would be signs of **cerebrovascular disease** – perhaps a history of a stroke or transient ischaemic attack, a history of having a heart attack, or the presence of risk factors for cerebrovascular disease (such as raised blood pressure, diabetes, raised cholesterol, atrial fibrillation, being overweight or

cerebrovascular disease

Any disease affecting an artery within the brain, or supplying blood to the brain.

smoking). These features of cerebrovascular disease, even if not already known, can be detected by physical examination (by taking a measure of blood pressure or the pulse) or by detecting raised cholesterol or raised sugar (indicative of diabetes) in a blood test.

A brain scan (either a CT or MRI scan) could reveal the presence of vascular changes in the brain – this can be either an area of stroke, where a wedge shaped area of the brain dies (see Plate 3), or by changes to the brain called 'white matter' changes (the white matter indicating damage to the colourings of nerve fibres in the brain). There can also be a combination of the two.

In someone with Alzheimer's disease, one might see particular shrinkage of the temporal lobe of the brain (the area associated with the preservation of memory). Sometimes, an ultrasound examination of the main arteries which supply blood to the brain (the carotid arteries) can show if there is narrowing of **arthrosclerotic plaques** in the carotid arteries.

A doctor will come to a decision about the type of dementia from which the patient is suffering by looking at all aspects of the history, examination and the results of investigations. A gradual onset of illness with no evidence of cerebrovascular disease will strongly favour Alzheimer's disease, while a history of stroke, associated with loss of memory, makes vascular dementia more likely, and the presence of intermittent confusion with signs of Parkinson's disease would likely lead to a diagnosis of Lewy body dementia.

arthrosclerotic plaques

A general term indicating the presence of the deposition of something abnormal – senile plaques can be seen deposited in the brain in between nerve fibres in Alzheimer's disease. Deposits of fat in arteries occur as part of the normal ageing process and predispose strokes, heart attacks and vascular dementia.

If any abnormal physical illness is found, for example a urinary tract infection, it should be treated in their own right.

Examination of a person with suspected dementia

✧ Mental state examination
    Depression
    Memory and associated features
✧ Physical examination
    Check for signs of a stroke
    Check for risk factors for a stroke
✧ Detailed tests of memory
    (neuropsychological tests)
✧ Investigations
    Blood tests
    Brain scan
    Chest X-ray
    Electrocardiogram
    Electroencephalogram.

my experience

I was referred to a memory clinic with memory loss and the nurse who saw me said I was to have a brain scan. I was immediately worried about this, because I don't like medical tests or investigations, and I was sure they were only suggesting this because they thought I had a brain tumour. I had to wait several weeks for the test, which did not help, and made me even more worried. I thought it was a specialist investigation, but I went to a general hospital and had the test in a general X-ray department, where people were getting normal X-rays for things like a broken leg. The staff were very kind and explained to me exactly what was going to happen. The two types of staff involved were radiologists (these are doctors who specialize in the use of X-rays to diagnose disease) and radiographers (the experts who carry out the tests).

I lay on a table with my head held still by a band across my forehead. This was to keep me still as moving my head would have meant the image on the scan would have been distorted. The table gradually moved back until my head was in the scanner. The radiologists were able to talk to me through a speaker in the room, and I was able to talk to them through a microphone. The test lasted about five or ten minutes but, to be honest, there was so much happening, and people were talking, that I did not really notice the time.

At the clinic, the doctors showed me the scan and the areas of my brain, which had shrunk slightly. There was no evidence that I had had a stroke, and no evidence of a brain tumour and it was concluded that the shrinkage of my brain was consistent with Alzheimer's disease.

CHAPTER

4

Treatments

Different approaches

Treatments for Alzheimer's disease can be divided into two categories. First, non-drug approaches, such as behaviour therapy and psychological support, and second, drug treatments. Each of these can be applied to the two main expressions of Alzheimer's disease – one, memory loss and, two, psychiatric symptoms and behavioural disturbances. For convenience sake, this section on the treatment of Alzheimer's disease will follow these divisions.

Non-drug treatment of psychiatric symptoms and behavioural disturbances

Many of the psychiatric symptoms and, later in the disease, the behavioural disturbances of

Alzheimer's disease, can be managed and treated very effectively without the need for drugs. The first thing that a doctor or nurse should do is to make sure that the patient and carer understand that the symptoms, generally speaking, arise as a consequence of the disease.

Memory loss

For example, if a person suffering from Alzheimer's disease misplaces a wallet or handbag, he or she may accuse someone else of moving it, or even having stolen it. A brief explanation that this can be seen as a natural response to forgetting where something is, can be helpful. A strategy, such as always putting a wallet or handbag or set of keys in one place, may be a solution.

Stubborn behaviour

If a sufferer has an idea which is firmly held, there is little point in trying to convince them that they are wrong and you are right. For example, some people with Alzheimer's disease say that their parents are still alive when they are dead. Sometimes people will try to get the person with Alzheimer's disease to say what age they are and then to calculate what age their parents would be if they were alive to prove they are wrong. This is an unhelpful approach and could be seen as serving only to humiliate the person. On the other hand, it is important not to agree with somebody, especially if their idea is clearly abnormal. The secret is probably never to completely agree or disagree but somehow take the middle ground.

Repetitive behaviour

It is also very common for people with Alzheimer's disease to repeat the same question again and again. It is best to try to avoid becoming irritable with the person and saying, 'You've asked me that question a hundred times'. They simply cannot remember. A technique which may be helpful in this situation is validation therapy. The principle behind this is to accept that recurrent themes emerge in repetitive questions or repetitive speech and that these themes reflect unmet needs or anxieties on the part of the person with Alzheimer's disease.

Often old memories of significant life experiences can emerge and dominate that person's reality for a period of time. Validation therapy allows us a way of entering into and sharing that person's reality to offer support and reassurance. The person who asks repeatedly, 'Where is mother?' may be reliving significant memories of their mother. Rather than reminding them that their mother has been dead for some years, which is a harsh approach, we can talk with them about their mother but always using the past tense. An opening comment such as, 'You're clearly thinking about your mother; she must have been a very important person in your life, so tell me about what she was like,' allows the person with Alzheimer's disease to express their concerns and anxieties. It allows them to talk about their mother and to remind themselves gradually that their mother indeed passed away some time ago.

Antisocial behaviour

Some behaviours such as aggression or screaming, when people are in the later stages of Alzheimer's disease, can be treated with what are called 'behavioural techniques'. In a sense it is a little like training children in that it is important to reinforce and give rewards when someone is good and not exhibiting bad behaviour rather than simply constantly telling them off when they are bad.

When someone becomes agitated or excited it is important to try to step back from the situation and to identify anything that seems to cause a particular behaviour, anything that seems to keep it happening and anything that seems to stop the behaviour. It may be that patterns will emerge which would be helpful in understanding and managing a particular symptom. For example, it is not uncommon for people with Alzheimer's disease to become agitated and excited in the evening. An example of this would be a woman suffering from Alzheimer's disease who begins to get agitated and worried when her husband, whom she is expecting home for his dinner, has not arrived.

Adopt a person-centred approach

Understanding the behaviour of the person with Alzheimer's disease rests almost exclusively upon trying to understand more about the person who is experiencing it. Adopting a person-centred approach reminds us that it is the unique individual who is important rather than the label or diagnosis they have acquired. Everyone with Alzheimer's disease has a unique life history, set of relationships, personality, habits and preferences. Understanding these can often help to determine the context of challenging behaviours and the messages that lie behind such behaviours.

The most important thing to remember when dealing with psychiatric symptoms or behavioural disturbances, and trying to manage them without drugs, is to understand that the person's actions are not under their own control and it is important to avoid getting angry and frustrated – however impossible this may seem! Also, and often contrary to popular belief, people with memory loss are able to respond to a kind, gentle and consistent approach and it is very important to try a strategy like this before resorting to drugs.

There are a number of other treatments which can help control agitation in people with severe Alzheimer's disease. A technique called 'the snoozelen' is a room where there are sounds, music, and things to touch and feel. This approach can decrease agitation in people with Alzheimer's disease. Likewise, there is some evidence that light therapy (where the person sits in front of a light box) can make people feel more calm.

In summary, try a non-drug approach to manage behavioural problems first, looking for explanations for the reasons behind behaviours, and avoid challenging the person with Alzheimer's disease even if they are obviously wrong. Do remember that the reactions of the person are often not under their own control.

Drug treatment of psychiatric symptoms and behavioural disturbances

If symptoms and behaviours are very distressing for the patient, or very distressing and disturbing for a carer, or the non-drug approaches have failed, it may be appropriate to consider a drug treatment. This is something that the patient's GP or a community psychiatric nurse can advise on.

There are a number of different types of drugs which may be helpful and a full list of drugs appears in Table 3 on pages 72–3.

Antidepressants

These treat symptoms of depression and can either be used if someone with a known dementia becomes depressed or if someone has a depressive illness and some symptoms of memory loss. There are a number of antidepressant drugs available and in terms of their effect on depression there is probably very little to choose between them. Some of the older drugs tend to have more side effects (for example, amytriptyline, which can give a dry mouth, constipation, blurred vision and dizziness), while some of the newer ones have fewer side effects (for example, sertraline, which can cause a tummy upset). Some antidepressants have a sedative effect but that can be an advantage if someone with depression is agitated or excited.

Neuroleptics

These are quite powerful drugs and are used to treat schizophrenia in younger people but can be very helpful in controlling aggression, agitation and delusions. Like the antidepressants, there are older and newer types. The older drugs, for example, chlorpromazine, thioridazine, promazine and haloperidol tend to have more side effects and people can get very stiff muscles and some of the symptoms of Parkinson's disease (these side effects are particularly marked in people with Lewy body dementia). Some of the newer neuroleptics (risperidone, olanzapine, Quetiapine or aripiprazole) tend to be less sedative and have

myth
Depression in older people cannot be treated.

fact
Depression in an older person may mimic the symptoms of dementia, and people with dementia are more prone to develop symptoms of depression. However, depressive symptoms can be treated quite effectively in older people, using drugs and, in some situations, psychological treatments (so-called 'talking therapies') can also be helpful. Depression can be a difficult illness to treat, but there is no reason to suppose that just because a person is older or has dementia, that treatment is ineffective.

fewer side effects. The regulatory agency which is part of the UK government that monitors the safety of drugs, the Committee on Safety of Medicines (CSM), issued a warning in March 2004 saying that risperidone and olanzapine could not be recommended for the treatment of agitation in people with dementia. The USA Food and Drug Administration (FDA) has recently come out with a warning for all the newer neuroleptics saying that there is an increased risk of stroke when they are prescribed to people with dementia. It stated that it was appropriate that they be prescribed when there were specific symptoms of psychosis and this had to be under the guidance of a specialist for as short a time as possible (weeks rather than months). However, if someone is very agitated and upset it still may be appropriate to prescribe one of the older drugs. Very occasionally in someone with Alzheimer's disease, the drugs can be given by an intramuscular injection. This is particularly useful if it is difficult for someone to take tablets but is something which should be considered only by a specialist.

Sedatives

These are drugs which generally make people more calm and can make them sleep. Examples are benzodiazapines (such as lorazepam, nitrazepam, temazepam and diazepam), chloramethiazole, and a number of sleeping agents (such as zopiclone). If there is no evidence that someone has delusions but is just slightly agitated, these drugs can be very effective. A drug called sodium valproate (which has been used in people with epilepsy) can also be useful in controlling agitation.

It has been suggested that if someone with Alzheimer's disease absolutely refuses to take drugs then it is justifiable to hide them in a drink or food and thus, effectively, give people drugs without them knowing it. This is an unethical and bad practice, although in very exceptional circumstances it may be justified for a short period of time for the safety and comfort of the patient. Drugs are generally available in a number of different forms such as a liquid, capsule or tablet and it is usually possible to find a formulation that suits each individual.

Q My father has Alzheimer's disease and was prescribed risperidone for agitation. The doctor then stopped it because he said there was an increased risk of stroke and he is a lot worse. What should I do?

A Risperidone is one of a group of drugs called the atypical antipsychotics. Trials have shown that this group of drugs is effective at reducing agitation in people with dementia. However, a further analysis of the studies showed that the risk of developing a stroke was three times higher in those taking these drugs compared to those on placebo in the trials and this is undoubtedly behind your doctor's withdrawal of the medication. However, in some people these drugs are extremely effective and the risks of prescribing it in an individual patient versus the benefit of prescribing them (in medicine, called the risk:benefit ratio) has to be considered carefully in each individual. That said, for people who respond very well to a drug, who do not have any of the risk factors for a stroke or transient ischaemic attack, the newer neuroleptics still have a valuable place in the management of dementia.

neuropsycho-logical features

Part of the expression of dementia characterized by amnesia (loss of memory), aphasia (problems understanding or expressing words), agnosia (failure to recognize people or objects) and apraxia (the inability to carry out tasks such as writing, dressing or using a knife and fork).

Non-drug treatment of memory loss and neuropsychological features

Memory retraining strategies

To date, most attempts to improve the memory of people with Alzheimer's disease have given poor results. It is not really surprising that there is a high degree of failure, as many of the methods used to teach people with Alzheimer's disease have been successful in groups of people free from dementia. One such method is the use of visual imagery which is often used with healthy older adults. This involves the creation of a 'picture' in the mind's eye that helps memory. For example, if a list of words is to be remembered, then it might be worth putting them together in a

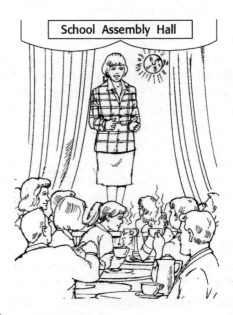

School Assembly Hall

Figure 3 Visual imagery.

'picture'. Say the words were: curtain, bell, coffee, school and parent (these are taken from a well used memory test) then a visual image might take the format shown in Figure 3.

Thus the picture for these five words could take the form of a parents' meeting at school. The head teacher of the *school* is standing on the stage with *curtains* talking to *parents* who are drinking *coffee* when the *bell* rings. The use of a technique such as this is often very effective at aiding memory in healthy people. However, when we try to use the same technique to help a person with Alzheimer's disease, they are more likely to fail. Why should this be? The reason is probably that this type of method is in actual fact quite difficult to perform. Even in healthy older adults, a good imagination is required in order to put all the items into the picture, and often it needs to be done quickly. Also it depends on the picture being remembered, so the visual memory, as we call it, needs to be performing fairly well. In Alzheimer's disease the abilities to concentrate, put together a picture quickly and to remember it can be poor, so this type of memory aid is not likely to be useful. The whole procedure is just too complex.

More encouragingly, there are some studies that have shown that people with Alzheimer's disease can, under certain conditions, improve their memory performance. Some of these techniques are described below.

Spaced retrieval technique

This is a teaching method that involves the recall of information at short intervals initially, with a gradual increase in the time interval. For example, if the task was to learn that the day of the week is

Friday, the person would be asked, maybe every three minutes, 'What day of the week is it today?' As gradual improvement is made, the time interval is increased from three to five minutes. If, however, they fail to get the answer right at five minutes the whole procedure reverts back to the three-minute interval, or whatever the time span was that enabled them to get the correct answer. If this does not lead to improvement, then the interval is halved. Accurate recall after a five- to ten-minute interval is deemed to be successful, according to the researchers who recommend this technique.

The advantages of the **spaced retrieval technique** is that it requires little effort from the person with Alzheimer's disease, and there is some evidence that often the learning becomes almost automatic and people can give the right answer without having to think about it. Also, probably because there is a high rate of success, people enjoy this method of training. Carers can be taught the basic principles of spaced retrieval and can incorporate it into their daily routines. People with mild and moderate Alzheimer's disease have been able to learn and recall information such as faces and names, where certain objects have been placed, the names of objects, and items such as days of the week, month, and date, etc.

spaced retrieval technique
A teaching method that involves the recall of information at short intervals initially, with a gradual increase in the time span.

Method of vanishing cues

This is a method that attempts to improve verbal memory skills by giving letters as clues to the required word. For example, if we wanted to teach the name JANE we might give the first three letters in the name:

vanishing cues
The attempts to improve verbal memory skills by giving letters/numbers as clues to a required answer.

J A N _

If the person is unable to produce the name, letters are progressively added until the correct name is attained. On the next training session one letter will be taken away. For example:

J A _ _

and so on until the learning progresses. If a person fails at any point, then letters are added to help them. This technique has been used with success in teaching people to learn names and occupations of staff members, addresses, telephone numbers and recognition of objects. In many cases the learning has been maintained for several weeks.

Errorless learning

This technique has been around for many years, although until very recently it has not been used with people with Alzheimer's disease. In the main, it has been helpful for teaching people with learning disabilities and people who have had a head injury, or brain disease of some kind. When people with Alzheimer's disease learn new information, they are often prone to failure. If we take an example of a typical learning scenario, such as learning a list of pairs using a traditional approach:

> friut – apple
> metal – iron
> baby – cries

After having read out the list of pairs, the experimenter would say, 'Which word goes with fruit?' If the person with Alzheimer's disease does not know the answer it is very tempting to encourage them to guess by saying, 'It's worth a try.' The problem with this is they probably know

errorless learning
A technique that prevents errors from being made during training.

the answer is a fruit and a guess might yield the wrong answer, so instead of 'fruit – apple' they may guess 'fruit – banana', which is obviously wrong, although a sensible guess. This wrong answer, however, is then almost locked into the brain and the person finds it difficult to correct it. Consequently, the next time they are asked, 'What word went with fruit?', they will inevitably reply 'banana'. This is what we call errorful learning.

Errorless learning is a method that prevents errors being made during training. It differs from errorful learning primarily because guessing is not encouraged. If a person does not know the right answer, they are given the answer, and therefore prevented from making errors. In the preliminary studies that have used this method there have been some good results. One study found that four participants were able to relearn face-name pairs, and recall personal information. In some of the cases the information had been retained over a period of six months.

Sensorimotor skills

Several researchers have found that the ability to perform certain simple skills are preserved in Alzheimer's disease. These might include tasks that have a 'motor' element to them, which means that they are usually tasks that involve a degree of manual dexterity, albeit at a fairly simple level. Such tasks might include combing the hair, washing, brushing the teeth, preparation of and eating meals, etc. The training would involve written and/or verbal instructions, and the task might be broken down into smaller goals so that each stage of the 'action' is taught before it is put together as a whole. Thus, the task is simplified and built up gradually. Similarly, motor skills that people have built up over a lifetime can often be maintained at some level, even in the moderate stage of the illness, and activities such as painting and playing a musical instrument can be stimulated with good results. Interestingly, it has been found that there may also be a knock-on effect of this type of training, in that 'untrained' skills can also improve spontaneously. It is almost as if stimulation and encouragement of certain motor activities improves other practical skills.

General techniques to improve memory

These tend to be used when people develop moderate to severe Alzheimer's disease. Before the anti-dementia drugs and recent advances in these techniques were considered to be the main treatment methods for improving memory in Alzheimer's disease.

Reality orientation

This can take two forms: classroom based or 24-hour reality orientation (RO) attempts to improve orientation and personal information.

Classroom-based RO: This takes place in a group situation, is of a fixed duration and is usually led by an occupational therapist. Demands on the group are minimal, and questions and comments are raised concerning areas such as weather, day, month, date and history, etc.

24-hour RO: This form of RO, as the name suggests, is meant to be ongoing. It involves the continued repetition of information (again focusing on weather, day, date, time, etc.) by staff, or anyone who is interacting with the person.

In effect, RO is a procedure whereby certain topics are constantly being brought up and practised. There is some evidence that this can help with aspects of memory, thinking and behaviour, but it has little benefits for the completion of practical tasks required for everyday life.

Reminiscence therapy

This focuses on the production of historical information that may stimulate long-term memories for the person with Alzheimer's disease. For example, photographs of a monarch's coronation, famous politicians or wartime scenes may evoke discussion and further memories. There is not a great deal of scientific evidence to support this therapy but some doctors do claim that there are benefits. In essence, this type of therapy is probably working because it is tapping into the long-term memory, which is usually better preserved than the short-term memory. This has implications for carers wanting to apply this type of therapy at home. Compiling a scrapbook with photographs, letters, etc. can form a personalized reminiscence book, focusing on interests, family and work that have been important to the person during his or her life. When communication abilities are lost, this type of tool can often help carers and relatives to interact, albeit at a reduced level.

External aids

External non-electronic memory aids such as diaries, calendars, signs and wipe-clean boards are useful aids for memory. In one study, a 'memory book' was produced which contained pictures of daily activities in conjunction with a clock face showing the right time for them to be carried out.

As electronic devices become more advanced, it seems appropriate to look at their usefulness for people with Alzheimer's disease. They can take over the role of prompting and reminding from the carer. For example, at a certain pre-determined time, an alarm will go off followed by a verbal message.

People with dementia can improve their memory performance but they need to be given help specifically tailored to their abilities. The type of assistance they require may differ from traditional teaching methods that are used for teaching healthy older adults.

Drug treatment of memory loss and neuropsychological features

This area has generated the most interest, and many drug companies are trying to develop medicines for the prevention and treatment of dementia, especially that caused by Alzheimer's disease.

Anticholinesterase drugs

These are commonly known as 'anti-dementia' drugs and work in the following way. The destruction of the brain by deposits of the abnormal protein found in Alzheimer's results in a chemical deficiency of a brain chemical (**neurotransmitter**) called 'acetylcholine'. Acetylcholine is made in the nerve cells and is used by these cells to communicate with each other. There is an enzyme that breaks down acetylcholine called 'cholinesterase'. If this enzyme is blocked, less of the acetylcholine is broken down and the net effect is to get a raised level. Research has shown that Alzheimer's patients can benefit greatly when given these drugs. Because

neurotransmitter
A chemical messenger in the brain which allows messages to be sent between brain cells (neurons).

anticholinesterase drugs
A new type of drug which improves the symptoms of Alzheimer's disease by raising the level of a neurotransmitter, acetylcholine, in the brain.

they act against the enzyme that breaks down acetylcholine they are called **anticholinesterase drugs**.

Q **What are the common side effects of the anti-dementia drugs?**

A The main side effects of the three drugs currently available (donepezil, rivastigmine and galantamine) are gastrointestinal side effects (indigestion, bowel disturbance, nausea and sickness), dizziness and agitation (some people can get over-excited and if the tablets are taken last thing at night people can have disturbed sleep and dreams). However, these side effects are relatively rare and short lived and probably affect about one person in 20. The drugs can also slow the heart rate.
Another drug, memantine, can have the side effect of causing agitation and people can also get symptoms of feeling dizzy and, more rarely, suffer from hallucinations (seeing or hearing things that aren't there). However, these are quite rare. For some reason which is not entirely clear, people on memantine seem to get urinary tract infections but these can usually be treated easily.

The first anti-dementia drug that was available was called tacrine. Although this produced significant benefit to people, its use was limited because in some people it damaged their liver. There are three drugs of this type that are now available (drugs usually have two names, a chemical name which describes the structure of the drug and a trade name which is the name the drug company gives it when it sold). Donepezil (trade name, Aricept®) was the first to be licensed in the UK. The next was rivastigmine (trade name, Exelon®). More recently there has been galantamine (trade name, Reminyl®) which comes from daffodils. These drugs have all been shown to be effective in improving objective tests of memory in people with mild to moderate Alzheimer's disease and also in improving global measures of well-being (this is an overall index, of whether a patient is better on a particular drug, and takes into account all the symptoms that a patient has and also includes the view of the carers).

The side effects of the drugs are minimal – dizziness and gastrointestinal upsets are the most common. There is evidence that the improvement can last for up to 12 months or perhaps even longer. There is also evidence that the sooner the drugs are started the better. While the drugs are currently only licensed for the treatment of mild to moderate Alzheimer's disease, some studies are underway looking at their effects in more severe illness.

Memantine

Memantine has recently been licensed in the UK for the treatment of moderately severe to severe Alzheimer's disease. It works in a different way from the other drugs because it blocks the effect of glutamate and another brain neurotransmitter which is actually present at a higher level in those suffering from Alzheimer's disease, and there is some evidence that these high levels are toxic to brain cells. It helps to stop the toxic effect of glutamate on one of the receptors on the nerve cell (called the NMDA receptor) but it sticks to this receptor relatively weakly – hence the drug's full name, a partial NMDA antagonist. Studies have been carried out in people with more severe Alzheimer's disease (some in nursing homes), which show that the drug could improve symptoms. There is some emerging evidence that combining memantine with the anticholinesterase

Q I've been prescribed Aricept®. I'm not getting any side effects. Does this mean it's not working?

A Every drug potentially has side effects and about one person in 20 who takes either Aricept® (donepezil), Reminyl® (galantamine) or Exelon® (rivastigmine) will get some side effects. However, the drug can still be effective even though you have no unwanted symptoms as a result of taking it.

My wife was diagnosed as having Alzheimer's disease about six months ago. Her memory had deteriorated about six months prior to that, and we went to see our GP, who referred us to the local memory clinic. They did a number of tests, including a CT brain scan, and then they told us that she was suffering from Alzheimer's disease. She was started on galantamine, and after a few weeks we began to notice that her memory was improving and she seemed more confident in things. She did get a few feelings of nausea for the first few days after treatment, but this soon wore off and it was helped when she took the tablet with food. She had a number of tests of her memory for the kinds of things she was doing round the house (they called it activities of daily living) as well as measures of how she was emotionally. They also asked me if I had noticed any difference and if our children were aware of any changes. The dose of galantamine was increased and she has now been on it for eighteen months. I really don't think she has got any worse in the last eighteen months or so.

donepezil can result in additional benefit but further research is needed to confirm this finding.

Oestrogens

These are given as part of hormone replacement therapy to women. There is some evidence from epidemiological (population) studies that taking oestrogen is protective against the development of Alzheimer's disease, although some more recent studies have suggested that it can increase the rates by which people get Alzheimer's disease. In people who already have dementia oestrogen is of no value in slowing down the progression of the disease.

Hydergine

This is a drug that improves blood circulation. Some people who are apathetic and withdrawn and have signs of Parkinsonism sometimes benefit from this drug which has an alerting effect.

Aspirin and other anti-inflammatory drugs

There is some evidence that taking aspirin and some other anti-inflammatory drugs is protective against the development of dementia. Specifically, aspirin is used in people with vascular dementia and who have had a stroke because there is good evidence that it can significantly reduce the chances of having a second stroke. There is less convincing evidence that if used in healthy people it can prevent someone having a heart attack or stroke, although there is increasing evidence that it may be helpful in this situation. Anti-inflammatory agents such as ibuprofen or brufen may have a protective effect against the development of Alzheimer's disease in epidemiological (population) studies. One study suggested that taking indomethacin, a type of anti-inflammatory drug, might help the symptoms of Alzheimer's disease but this is only one study and the results have not been replicated. It would be very unwise to take any anti-inflammatory drug or aspirin (which can cause ulcers and potentially severe bleeding in the stomach and upper intestine) without specialist advice from a doctor.

Gingko biloba

Some studies have suggested that gingko biloba can improve memory and concentration but others have produced negative results. Some people describe improvements while taking gingko biloba but there is not enough evidence to recommend its use.

Anti-oxidants

Vitamin E may delay the progression of Alzheimer's disease and some people take it for its protective action. However, it is worth mentioning that a recent study suggested that vitamin E was ineffective at halting the progression from mild cognitive impairment to Alzheimer's disease. Vitamin E removes substances called 'free radicals' which can cause nerve cell damage. This is similar to the effect of red wine which some believe is protective against the development of Alzheimer's disease.

Statins

Statins are drugs which are used to lower the level of cholesterol in the blood. As high cholesterol has been associated with heart attacks and strokes, testing of cholesterol is very widely available (it is even available in some chemists). Statins are now becoming much more widely prescribed. There is some evidence from epidemiological (population) studies that taking a statin reduces the chances of getting Alzheimer's disease. The exact reason for this is not known, but it does seem to be a little more complicated than the obvious one, i.e. taking a statin reduces the risk of vascular disease and therefore the risk of Alzheimer's disease. People with dementia should have their cholesterol checked as part of a general medical examination, and if the cholesterol is high (after, for example, diet has been tried) then drugs should be prescribed. They are not without side effects, and their prescription purely to prevent Alzheimer's disease is not justified, but that may be an added benefit for those who are taking them anyway.

myth
The Alzheimer's vaccine can stop the process of Alzheimer's disease.

fact
The vaccine, when it was introduced, was hailed as a great step forward because it had the potential to dissolve the abnormal proteins which are laid down in the brain in Alzheimer's disease. However, the vaccine had quite bad side effects and some people got an inflammation of the brain (encephalitis). Much more work needs to be done to find out the cause of that and to develop a similar vaccine that does not have these effects.

Vaccine

The vaccine has been developed to try to get rid of the abnormal protein which is deposited in the brains of people with Alzheimer's disease by setting up an immune reaction against the protein (in a similar way that if you have a cold, the body's own defence mechanism makes up antibodies to get rid of the infection). Antibodies created by having the vaccine could, theoretically, remove the abnormal protein and improve the symptoms of Alzheimer's disease. However, sadly, the vaccine has many side effects, especially a general inflammation of the brain which tragically, in some circumstances, led to death. More work is being done on the vaccine to see if the benefits can outweigh the disadvantages but there is no immediate prospect of a vaccine being available for Alzheimer's disease.

Prevention of dementia

The question is often asked whether it is possible to prevent Alzheimer's disease. There are well-established risk factors for vascular dementia and some of these have also emerged as being risk factors for Alzheimer's disease. These include raised blood pressure, raised cholesterol, a deficiency of folic acid (often signalled by an increase in homocysteine in the blood), smoking, atrial fibrillation (an abnormal beating of the heart which predisposes to clots in the heart which can travel up the blood vessels into the brain) and obesity. There is also good evidence to show that regular physical exercise and mental activity can protect against Alzheimer's disease. A number of studies have shown that moderate alcohol intake can be protective against cardiovascular disease (heart attacks) and cerebrovascular disease (strokes) as well as dementia. Red wine is the most studied drink and there is biochemical evidence to suggest that specific antioxidant activity in red wine may protect blood vessels from damage.

The evidence is not sufficiently great to recommend one or all of these strategies for the prevention of dementia, but common sense dictates that the control of risk factors has benefits not only in terms of dementia but also with regard to strokes and blood pressure and that it is sensible to take reasonable and appropriate care of oneself – 'moderation in all things'.

Some drugs are said to have a beneficial effect. Aspirin may reduce the risk of strokes and heart attacks and there is some evidence to suggest that it may be good for the prevention of dementia. Oestrogens, once thought to be preventive against dementia, may now actually increase the risk in older women.

Table 2 Drugs used to treat dementia.

ANTIDEPRESSANTS

Chemical name	Trade name	Used for
Amitriptyline	Lentizol®	Depression
Chlormipramine	Anafranil®	Depression
Dothiepin	Prothiedin®	Depression
Imipramine	Tofranil®	Depression
Lofepramine	Gamanil®	Depression
Trazodone	Molipaxin®	Depression/agitation
Moclobinide	Manorex®	Depression
Citalopram	Cipramil®	Depression
Fluoxetine	Prozac®	Depression
Fluvoxamine	Faverin®	Depression
Paroxetine	Seroxat®	Depression
Sertraline	Lustral®	Depression
Mirtazapine	Zipin®	Depression
Nefazodone	Dutonin®	Depression
Venlafaxine	Efexor®	Depression

NEUROLEPTICS

Chemical name	Trade name	Used for
Chlorpromazine	Largactil®	Aggression/agitation/psychosis
Haloperidol	Haldol®, Serenance®, Dozic®	Aggression/agitation/psychosis
Promazine	Sparine®	Aggression/agitation/psychosis
Thioridazine	Melleril®	Aggression/agitation/psychosis
Trifluoperazine	Stelazine®	Psychosis
Olanzapine	Zyprexa®	Psychosis/agitation
Risperidone	Risperdal®	Psychosis/agitation
Quetiapine	Seroquel®	Psychosis/agitation

SEDATIVES

Chemical	Trade name	Used for
Nitrazepam	Mogadon®	Sedation
Temazepam	Temazepam®	Sleeplessness
Lorazepam	Ativan®	Sedation
Diazepam	Valium®, Valclair®	Sedation
Zolpadine	Stilnoct®	Sleeplessness
Zopiclone	Zimovane®	Sleeplessness
Chloral hydrate	Welldorm®	Sleeplessness
Chlormathiazole	Heminevrin®	Agitation
Sodium valporate	Epilim®	Agitation

Table 2 continued

ANTICHOLINESTERASE DRUGS		
Chemical	**Trade name**	**Used for**
Donepezil	Aricept®	To improve memory and behaviour
Rivastigmine	Exelon®	To improve memory and behaviour
Galantamine	Reminyl®	To improve memory and behaviour

GLUTAMATERGIC DRUG		
Chemical	**Trade name**	**Used for**
Memantine	Ebixa®	To improve memory and behaviour

In the prevention of dementia it is important to remember a few key points:

◇ Drugs are available which can help reverse the memory problems in early Alzheimer's disease

◇ They are not a cure

◇ They are not effective in everyone

◇ Vitamin E, in large doses, can be helpful in slowing the progression of Alzheimer's disease

◇ Aspirin can be helpful in preventing strokes

◇ There is no scientific evidence that gingko biloba is effective against dementia

◇ Always consult your doctor before taking anything you can buy without a prescription.

Q Is there any reason why someone with Alzheimer's disease could not be prescribed one of the anticholinesterase drugs?

A The most common reason is if the heart rate is very low (usually less than 50 beats a minute) or if there is evidence of a blockage to the electrical activity of the heart (heart block). This is because the drugs tend to slow the heart down and so if the heart rate is very slow anyway or there is a problem with the rhythm of the heart, it is best to avoid the drugs altogether.

CHAPTER

5

The experience of dementia

The impact on the patient

The experience of Alzheimer's disease is frequently described as a journey. The sufferer starts the journey alone with the personal recognition that there is a change in their abilities or memory performance. As the changes progress, others join in to offer support or companionship. Some companions on the journey travel only a short distance, perhaps offering specific services at specific times, while others go the full distance. This section is about this journey and the impact that Alzheimer's disease can have upon those who are challenged to undertake it.

Whatever the severity of the symptoms of Alzheimer's disease, they will always have an impact upon the person who experiences them and this impact will usually be evident to others because of changes in the mood or behaviour of the person with Alzheimer's.

All of the symptoms of Alzheimer's are being brought about by the illness or disability that the person is experiencing. Some of them, for instance changes in mood or behaviour such as agitation or depression, may also occur as a direct consequence of the way in which the person with Alzheimer's feels about him or herself or reacts to the care that others may offer. It is these specific changes that we will discuss in this section.

Mild dementia

In the early stages of Alzheimer's disease the person will experience mild and often very subtle changes. These changes will always represent a change to that person's previous way of performing and will be evident to that person. At first they may be so mild as to generate amusement rather than concern and even as they progress, the sufferer and those around him or her, may attempt to disregard them as being the result of age, stress or a busy lifestyle.

The 'hidden phase'

This initial stage is often referred to as the **'hidden phase' of a dementia**, as the changes represent difficulties rather than problems and may not be obvious to others or may easily be dismissed. However, as they progress a little further, amusement or indifference begins to give way to concern and the person with Alzheimer's disease, or a concerned relative, may seek advice from the family doctor.

During the hidden phase of dementia even mild and subtle changes in performance will have a psychological impact upon the person who

'hidden phase' of dementia
A very mild and subtle change in memory which may not be regarded as abnormal.

myth

People with dementia do not get anxious.

fact

Anxiety is a common symptom in Alzheimer's disease as the person becomes aware of deteriorating memory and begins to withdraw from social situations in the fear that they will embarrass themselves.

experiences them. The person with Alzheimer's disease is aware of the changing nature of their intellectual performance and may begin to become anxious, and this anxiety will be expressed through their behaviour. They may complain more of mild physical problems such as indigestion or headaches, they may lose concentration easily and become less efficient at work or home, they may start to withdraw from certain activities which are becoming challenging and this may include social activities so it appears that the person is becoming withdrawn or disinterested. Alongside this worry about their abilities or performance, the affected person may also become frustrated with themselves when they are unable to remember something or are unable to do something which they used to find so easy.

Q I lost my car keys last week. Does that mean I am developing Alzheimer's disease?

A No, not in itself. Losing things and forgetting people's names is a common thing and happens as people get older, as well as when people are under stress. An isolated incident is of no significance. If it begins to happen more often, if you forget something important or significant (for example, a hospital appointment or someone's birthday), then that might suggest you should go to your doctor for some advice. It is hard to say how often these things should happen before you should get worried, but generally, if they are occurring once a fortnight, or certainly once a week, it might be a good idea to consult your doctor. The most important warning signs of Alzheimer's disease are its progression and the speed of progression. If you notice these incidents of forgetfulness becoming more frequent, consult your doctor.

This frustration will lead to impatience and irritability and will also result in outbursts of anger, usually directed at inanimate objects or at themselves and then at the closest person to them, a husband or wife, for example, who may be verbally abused or blamed for what is happening. These two symptoms of anxiety and frustration are interconnected and exacerbate each other, bringing about a vicious circle; the more frustrated the person gets the harder it becomes to remember something, the harder it is to remember something the more anxious they become, the more anxious they become the harder it is to remember something, and the cycle continues.

An outcome of this cyclical process, and the reinforcement of failure it may bring about, may well be for the person with Alzheimer's disease to become depressed. During the hidden phase of dementia the onset of memory problems may be dismissed as being the consequence of depression and certainly there are some similarities between the symptoms of both with apathy, social withdrawal and loss of interest being commonly witnessed. In the later stages of Alzheimer's disease, signs of depression are frequently regarded as being the exacerbation of the dementing illness.

What is often forgotten is that Alzheimer's disease and depression are not mutually exclusive and can frequently co-exist. Failure to recognize the symptoms of Alzheimer's disease and dismiss them as depression acts to prolong the 'hidden phase', and failure to recognize depressive symptoms following a diagnosis of Alzheimer's disease serves to deny that person effective treatment.

myth

The person with dementia does not know what is happening to them.

fact

In the early stages, dementia is a frightening experience and certainly perplexing to the individual and that may explain some symptoms such as agitation, crying or restlessness.

myth

I have got memory loss, but someone said I might be depressed as well.

fact

There are many symptoms of depression. One symptom, of course, is feeling depressed. Other symptoms include fatigue and tiredness, loss of enjoyment or loss of pleasure in things, poor appetite and weight loss, feelings of guilt, insomnia or hypersomnia (sleeping too little or sleeping too much), irritability, poor concentration, a feeling of dread for the future, and suicidal ideas. The diagnosis of depression is complex, and if you are in any doubt you should seek the advice of your doctor.

The 'apparent phase'

At this point, with increasing severity of symptoms, we now start to enter the so-called **'apparent phase' of dementia**, the period of time when others become both aware of and concerned by the presence of memory problems in the person with dementia and the changes in mood and behaviour which they are causing. Very often there are common experiences, which occur and propel us forward into the apparent phase, these include:

✧ Becoming very repetitive in conversation or making frequent and repetitive phone calls to family members

✧ Having very little recall of significant current events involving the family and becoming angry when asked about them

✧ Getting lost when driving in a familiar place or frequently losing the car

✧ Getting dressed and leaving for work when that person has been retired for a number of years

✧ Becoming unable to use familiar household appliances such as a kettle or an electric razor and becoming frustrated and impatient when attempting to

✧ Becoming disoriented to time and standing outside shops or other places during the night or early hours of the morning (Disorientation may be particularly marked when the person is in unfamiliar surroundings, for example, on holiday)

✧ Forgetting to turn off the cooker or other appliances.

Even though the person is now entering a new phase of the dementing illness and even though problems are becoming apparent to others it does not necessarily follow that a diagnosis of dementia will now be made. Sometimes the changes from a clinical perspective may be so mild as to not raise a suspicion of dementia and the family doctor may not feel that referral to a specialist service is required. Eventually, however, the dementing illness progresses and the frequency and severity of symptoms increases to the point at which it is readily apparent to all that a problem exists.

Q **My father has just been diagnosed as having Alzheimer's disease, having had the symptoms for three years. How quickly will he get worse?**

A There is a wide variation in how quickly people with Alzheimer's disease deteriorate but, unfortunately, they all do. Broadly speaking, the illness can last from anything between five and 20 years. Generally, people who are younger (say someone who gets Alzheimer's disease at aged 60 as opposed to aged 80) would tend to have a more rapid decline and the presence of some features, such as a language problems early in the course of the illness, may also be associated with a more rapid decline, as are the presence of Parkinsonian symptoms (muscle stiffness, tremor, tremor with walking, an expressionless face and seborrhea (an excess secretion of oil by the skin giving the impression of sweating).

Moderate dementia

For most of this period the person with Alzheimer's disease will be experiencing moderate to moderately severe symptoms of their illness. At this stage the person is no longer having memory difficulties but problems, and these problems are making a significant impact upon their everyday life. Common problems, which would suggest moderate dementia, could include:

✧ No longer recalling your address
✧ Getting lost frequently in very familiar places including own home
✧ No longer recognizing familiar objects such as a telephone
✧ Losing track within a sentence and not being able to finish it
✧ Beginning to lose the understanding of other's speech
✧ Beginning to have difficulty talking
✧ Inability to make decisions or solve problems
✧ Becoming dependent upon others for cooking or shopping.

These problems suggest that the person with Alzheimer's disease is becoming more disabled by their illness and this deterioration can be witnessed through changes in their mood and behaviour.

Some of the most evident changes will reflect the growing detachment from reality that the person with Alzheimer's disease is experiencing. This sense of disorientation is itself a progressive phenomenon, causing that person to become increasingly uncertain, unsure and perplexed by everyday life. The classic presentation of disorientation is for it to occur in a cumulative fashion and the extent of the uncertainty being suggestive of the severity of that person's dementia. Commonly experienced disorientations, in roughly the order they occur, are:

✧ To date (tends to happen first)
✧ To day of the week
✧ To month
✧ To year
✧ To season

myth
Disorientation to place occurs earlier than disorientation to time.

fact
Generally speaking, people become disorientated to time first – they forget the date, then the day of the week, then the month, then the year, then the season, and then they become disorientated to place. Not immediately knowing the date is a common everyday experience. Also, when an elderly person is in hospital it is quite easy to lose track of time.

✧ To place
✧ To other's identities
✧ To personal identity.

The experience of becoming progressively disoriented or detached from reality is frequently termed 'confusion' but such a bland term does little to convey the often frightening nature of becoming suspended in a reality which is no longer familiar or which cannot be understood. By the time moderate dementia has taken hold, the level of disorientation will have moved on from affecting time relationships, to now affecting relationships to place and awareness of other's identities. Not surprisingly, a state in which the person is markedly distanced from our understanding of reality will have a significant impact upon their mood and behaviour.

Feeling uncertain around other people or in unfamiliar environments may make that person reluctant to venture away from home, where they will feel safer and more in control. This may be perceived as that person becoming less sociable or less motivated to do new things or to visit new places. This social reluctance will be worsened if that person retains an insight into their problems with memory and possibly speech, as they will experience embarrassment or feel challenged by the expectations of social activity.

The focus of everyday life therefore starts to become reduced as facets of that everyday life become challenging and anxiety provoking. Life may now appear to revolve almost exclusively around the person's symptoms or needs and it will seem that they have become selfish or indifferent to the needs of others. In reality, the disabilities brought about by Alzheimer's disease are so dominant that the person experiencing them will find attempts at comprehending or appreciating others' needs as much of a challenge as trying to understand life in general. Mental resources will be diminished and taking up these challenges will be exhausting and, as a consequence, the person's attention and energy is devoted to making sense of life.

Acting to further confound this situation are the other facets of Alzheimer's disease and, in particular, difficulties with communication. A number of speech and language symptoms may occur and these include:

✧ Word finding problems
✧ Naming difficulties
✧ Use of inappropriate words
✧ Repetition
✧ Misunderstanding of others' speech.

Being suspended in a reality, different from our own, which is possibly frightening, certainly perplexing, and not being able to verbally communicate this bewilderment serves to further isolate the person with dementia. Alternative means of communication may well develop to enable the person to articulate these feelings of distress, or needs which are not being met, and commonly behaviour may be the method of communication. Often this behaviour is termed problematic and may include:

✧ Aggression
✧ Shouting or screaming
✧ Crying
✧ Wandering
✧ Agitation
✧ Restlessness.

They may be better described as challenging behaviours because we are being challenged to understand the message that is being conveyed.

Some people with Alzheimer's disease may become aggressive to others and this may be an attempt to communicate fear, anxiety, uncertainty or pain. Some may shout or scream as a response to under-stimulation, to boredom or frustration. Crying may indicate depression and wandering may suggest that memories of a previously purposeful activity have resurfaced or that the person is trying to find something or distance themselves from negative feelings by trying to walk away from them.

A significant change in the person with moderate dementia, expressed through their behaviour, is the changing nature of that person's ability to function in day-to-day activities. Dementia robs people of their ability to function in their normal everyday manner. This is again progressive and, as functioning becomes impaired, others need to assist and to assume a greater degree of responsibility.

For the person with Alzheimer's disease who retains some insight, this dependency upon others will further induce feelings of distress, frustration, worthlessness and anger. Where insight has been lost the person with Alzheimer's disease may angrily reject or resist the essential care of others.

Severe dementia

The nature of dementia is for problems with memory and functioning to progress to the point at which that person becomes very significantly disabled and very highly dependent upon others. The final severest and terminal stage of all dementias occurs at the very end of the illness which has brought about the dementia and represents the very end of what may have been an arduous journey.

In this stage the person with dementia will appear to be very changed from when they developed mild difficulties and commenced the journey. Common symptoms will now include:

✧ No noticeable memory ability
✧ No functional ability
✧ A high level of dependency upon others
✧ Incontinence
✧ No effective communication ability
✧ Sporadic episodic challenging behaviours.

The person with severe dementia is now severely affected by their illness and will eventually die as even the basic ability of the body to fight infections or to regulate normal functioning is now affected. This can be a traumatic stage of the illness for the carer, particularly as it is difficult to understand what the person with dementia is experiencing and the realization that the companion on that long journey no longer shares any recognition or memory of the experience.

The impact on others

Alzheimer's disease naturally has an impact upon the person affected by it, but others who have a relationship with them may often be as affected in terms of their emotions and behaviour. Usually these other people will have a significant relationship with the person with Alzheimer's such as a close family member or friend, but sometimes they may have a less significant relationship, such as a work colleague or occasional acquaintance. The degree to which these other people are affected by the sufferer's difficulties depends upon three closely related factors:

- ✧ The nature of the relationship
- ✧ The severity of the person's difficulties
- ✧ The way in which the person responds to their difficulties.

The closer a person is to someone experiencing memory impairments, the more they will feel them impact upon themselves and their life. In terms of relationships, it can be any of the following:

- ✧ Spouse or partner
- ✧ Dependant or adult offspring
- ✧ Parent
- ✧ Sibling
- ✧ Friend
- ✧ Work colleague or employee
- ✧ Social acquaintance
- ✧ Neighbour.

Although we would traditionally regard the first few on the list as being examples of important relationships, it is necessary to recognize that any of the above can constitute a significant relationship.

In general terms, a significant relationship would imply that some part of everyday life involves the sufferer and that a strong emotional bond exists between both people. In many couples there will be a mutual responsibility for decision making, problem solving or planning alongside a relationship built upon affection, trust and understanding and, to a lesser extent, other significant relationships are built upon the same foundations.

Memory impairment of whatever severity acts to erode these foundations and to make those relationships fragile and vulnerable to change for the worse. In the case of a progressive illness, such as Alzheimer's disease, it may be that part of the progression is for some relationships to end, some to change and some to become more difficult in much the same way as companions on the journey into dementia come and go.

As memory performance declines, so everyday life becomes disrupted. In mild dementia such disruption may be fairly minimal, while in moderate or severe impairment it may be catastrophic. A large part of this disruption occurs because of the fact that whatever the relationship, there will always be a greater responsibility placed upon the person who does not have memory impairment. In memory impairments which persist or progress, then this devolving of responsibility will occur more and more, leading to a distinct inequality in the relationship. Shared activities will cease to be shared and the non-sufferer will be forced to assume a more dominant role, which may in itself represent a significant change in that relationship.

In mild memory loss the person may need to be reminded about appointments, they may need to be left written notes or the non-sufferer may need to start taking sole responsibility for important things such as paying bills. As the impairments progress and become more severe, the non-sufferer may have to assume almost total responsibility for household management, for driving or organizing transport and may even need to remind the sufferer about personal care, such as having a bath or wearing clean clothes.

Alongside the severity of the impairment, it is also important to remember the toll that these problems levy on the sufferer because how they react to them will often dictate how the non-sufferer reacts and what changes occur within the relationship. The impact on the sufferer has been discussed previously but for the purposes of this section their reaction can be considered in fairly simplistic terms of either positive or negative.

Positive and negative reactions of the sufferer

A positive reaction would usually occur in the early stages of dementia and could encompass a willingness to seek help or to develop routines which help to minimize the difficulties and a verbal appreciation to the non-sufferer for the extra work that they may have to do.

A negative approach could occur at any level of severity and would encompass such things as denying that a problem exists, readily blaming others when things are forgotten or becoming angry or abusive. In cases of dementia we can also include challenging behaviours or psychiatric symptoms, such as hallucinations or delusions, if they occur, as negative factors. Having said this, it is crucial to also say that we should not blame those sufferers who do react in a negative way, as often this may well be simply a further symptom over which they have no control.

A positive reaction in the sufferer will make it easier for the non-sufferer to adopt a positive attitude, while a negative reaction will worsen the experience for the non-sufferer and will serve to

Q **If a person with Alzheimer's disease is being aggressive because they think someone has come into the house to steal their possessions, are they aware of what they are saying?**

A People with dementia can have a number of what others would call 'abnormal ideas' because of problems with memory. This can be an everyday experience. For example, if we lose or misplace something, we may think that somebody has stolen it. When people with Alzheimer's disease have the delusion that someone has stolen their things, that is something that they really believe, and nothing can argue them out of it. That is the definition of a delusion, i.e. a fixed false belief. In those circumstances, the person is acting on what they truly believe and so, for them, they are not doing anything unusual.

rapidly challenge his or her own emotional health. The key to responding positively to the experience of dementia is working together as a partnership, being honest and openly addressing the problems and challenges that arise.

To do so, it is important to understand that the non-sufferer will be affected physically and emotionally by the sufferer's impairments, and when considering the commonest ways in which mood or behaviour may change it is also important to remember that:

✧ The closer the relationship to the sufferer, the greater the changes on the non-sufferer's mood and behaviour
✧ A negative reaction in the sufferer will increase the severity of the changes in the non-sufferer's mood and behaviour.

Changes to the non-sufferer's own mood and behaviour may occur in response to the impairments at any level of severity. There is often, however, a commonly occurring cumulative process, which means that the changes brought about by mild impairments are also brought about by moderate impairments and then extra ones can also occur. It may therefore be useful to consider the changes that can happen to the non-sufferer at each level of severity.

Mild memory impairments

✧ Irritation
✧ Frustration
✧ Anger
✧ Impatience
✧ Being argumentative

- ✧ Being amused
- ✧ Feeling unloved
- ✧ Feeling under appreciated.

Moderate memory impairments

- ✧ All of the above but to a greater extent
- ✧ No longer feeling amused
- ✧ Worried or anxious that a problem exists
- ✧ Assuming greater responsibility
- ✧ Loss of confidence in the sufferer
- ✧ Dislike of the sufferer
- ✧ Feeling tearful or upset
- ✧ Lacking concentration
- ✧ Experiencing mild memory difficulty
- ✧ Suffering from mild depression.

Severe memory impairments

- ✧ All of the above but to a greater extent
- ✧ Feelings of isolation
- ✧ Exhaustion
- ✧ Experiencing physical complaints
- ✧ Stress
- ✧ Guilt.

As well as understanding that changes can occur, it is also crucial to remember that carers of people with dementia do cope and do survive the journey they have embarked upon. Studies of carers have demonstrated the positive ways in which they have been able to cope. Some of the common methods have included:

- ✧ Blaming the illness, not the person affected by it
- ✧ Taking life one day at a time
- ✧ Trying to see the funny side of things
- ✧ Preserving a little bit of time for yourself

◇ Having an interest outside of caring
◇ Sharing feelings of anger and resentment openly with others.

All of these positive ways of coping seem to share an ability to keep a certain perspective on things but this is difficult to achieve since the non-sufferer is, after all, not a neutral observer. It is very easy to succumb to ways of coping and behaving which carers have described as being unhelpful. Very common reasons are not accepting that there is a problem and trying to deny or ignore its real presence and refusing offers of help from others.

It is important to understand that if the experience of dementia is a journey then it is going to be difficult and at times exhausting. Along the way there will, without doubt, come a point when you can no longer give the level of care that is required. Handing over care for an hour, a day, and a weekend, or permanently will never be easy and you will feel guilty, humiliated and ashamed or as if you have betrayed that person.

The reality is that the impact of the illness is powerful and often the promise, made in the early days after diagnosis, never to admit the person with dementia into care is one that can rarely be kept. If the carer accepts this, and is open about plans early on, it will do something to ameliorate the feelings they will experience.

Very many carers have described the positive impact that dementia brings. Some liken the post-diagnostic feeling to one of comrades in adversity and for many this strengthens the emotional ties underpinning their relationship. Others have described caring as giving them an opportunity to express, in a very practical way, their gratitude for what may have been a long and loving relationship. Some carers have described how responding to the challenging behaviours of dementia, through tact, gentleness and sensitivity, have presented an opportunity to engage in courting that person again with displays of love, attentiveness and attempts to make that person happy.

Finally it would appear that making a positive adjustment to the experience of dementia rests upon the following:

✧ Knowing and understanding the diagnosis
✧ Openly sharing problems and concerns
✧ Mutually planning for the future
✧ Accepting help when it is offered.

Driving and dementia

There is now emerging evidence that people with Alzheimer's disease have an impaired ability to drive – particularly where complex judgements have to be made which take into account a number of stimuli, for example, at road junctions. Obviously, by the time someone has deteriorated to the extent that they get lost when driving, their ability to handle a car is severely compromised. However, there is evidence to suggest that people with early Alzheimer's disease actually have less claims and cause fewer accidents than young men, and so any issue about driving in dementia has to be discussed in terms of risk to the individual rather than a public safety campaign.

It is never going to be easy for someone with developing dementia or Alzheimer's disease who has been driving for, say, 40 years, to be told that they are no longer capable of driving a car. People

myth
Everyone who receives a diagnosis of Alzheimer's disease has to give up driving.

fact
People with very mild dementia can still drive but that decision has to be made by the DVLA – it is not down to your doctor to decide whether you are able to drive or not. If you have been given a diagnosis of Alzheimer's disease, you are under a legal obligation to tell the DVLA (if you don't your insurance may not be valid). They then send a specialist form, via your GP, to fill in and then come to a decision as to whether you should drive or not.

invariably suggest that they are very safe drivers and only take the car on short journeys, but that is immaterial. The sufferer (and their spouse) is under an obligation to inform the Driving and Vehicle Licensing Agency (DVLA) that a condition (dementia and/or Alzheimer's disease) has been diagnosed which may affect their ability to drive. If a carer is very concerned about someone with dementia driving, they should mention it to their doctor in confidence.

The DVLA has a standard form, which they send to the doctor involved. The doctor, with the permission of the patient, provides information to the DVLA who then make a judgement on that person's ability to drive. Some people appeal against a decision (in practice, always a decision to revoke a licence) and they do have the ability to have a re-test. Interestingly, the doctor is asked to sign something to allow the person to have driving lessons for a day to allow them to undertake a re-test. In practice, a licence would only be renewed for a period of a year and then reviewed and it is probably safe to say that once a diagnosis of Alzheimer's disease has been made, a person's driving days are drawing to a close.

If a person, understandably, continues to insist on driving, then the doctor may, in certain circumstances, tell the DVLA if he or she is concerned with public safety. However, this is not something which is done lightly and usually only happens after prolonged negotiation between the patient, the doctor and their family. It is not unknown for spouses to have to hide car keys or even disable the car to stop the person from driving. In addition to this, although not a problem in the UK at present, there are a large number of older people in the USA who hold private pilot licences and this is an emerging issue for them.

CHAPTER

6

Services

Different types of care

A range of services is available to people suffering from Alzheimer's disease and, broadly speaking, the way in which a patient presenting with symptoms suggestive of Alzheimer's disease goes through the system, from primary care to specialist services (sometimes known as a 'care pathway'), is similar across the UK. There are slight differences depending on where you live and on what services are available locally but the main provision is similar.

General practice

Your GP is always the first point of contact. This contact can be carried out in several different ways. A person can go to their GP complaining of memory problems, for example, a concern about forgetting someone's name, missing an

fact

General practitioners, generally speaking, do not have access to the specialist diagnostic procedures to diagnose Alzheimer's disease. However, they are in the unique position of knowing the person and their family and will carry out blood tests. With a comprehensive referral, by the time a person is seen at a memory clinic, about 80% of the diagnostic work is usually done. At the time of writing, general practitioners cannot start treatment with anti-dementia drugs. This is done by a specialist, but follow-up is increasingly being done in primary care (general practice).

appointment or losing a set of keys. Your GP, generally speaking, is the doctor who knows you best and has access to all your records. They are in the best position to make an initial judgement as to the cause of your memory problems and will be able to take into account your past history, any current medical or surgical conditions you have, what drugs you are taking and when they were started.

Although GPs tend to have less time with patients for an initial consultation than a hospital specialist, a great deal of information can be gathered in that initial session. Your GP may arrange to see you again, may ask to see members of your family, may order some investigations such as blood tests or, even after one consultation, may be confident enough to refer you for a specialist assessment.

Your GP may carry out a structured examination of your memory with a test such as the Mini Mental State Examination or the Abbreviated Mental Test Score. These are shown in Tables 3 and 4 opposite and on page 96 below.

The second way a person with dementia could come to the attention of their GP is when a friend or relative alerts their doctor to the fact that they are worried about the person's memory. Typically, it might be a person's son or daughter who has noticed a decline in their parent's memory and, sometimes after some persuasion, the older person will go along for an assessment. In broad terms, the assessment follows the pattern described above although there needs to be a little more tact involved if it is clear that the older person is not there of their own free will. It may be a district nurse or health visitor who brings a memory problem to the attention of a GP.

Table 3 Mini Mental State Examination.

MMSE Sample Items

1 Orientation to Time
   "What is the date?"

2 Registration
   "Listen carefully. I am going to say three words. You say them back after I stop.
   Ready? Here they are . . .

   HOUSE (pause),
   CAR (pause),
   LAKE (pause).

   Now repeat those words back to me."

   [Repeat up to 5 times, but score only the first trial.]

3 Naming
   "What is this?"
   [Point to a pencil or pen.]

4 Reading
   "Please read this and do what it says."
   [Show examinee the words on the stimulus form.]
   CLOSE YOUR EYES

Table 4 Abbreviated Mental Test Score.

This is a quick and easy test that can be used in the consultation.

		EACH QUESTION SCORES ONE POINT
1	Age	☐
2	Time to nearest hour	☐
3	An address – for example 42 West Street – to be repeated by the patient at the end of the test	☐
4	Year	☐
5	Name of hospital, residential institution or home address, depending on where the patient is situated	☐
6	Recognition of two persons – for example, doctor, nurse, home help, etc.	☐
7	Date of birth	☐
8	Year First World War started	☐
9	Name of present monarch	☐
10	Count backwards from 20 to 1	☐
	Total score	

A SCORE OF LESS THAN SIX SUGGESTS DEMENTIA

In addition to complaints of memory loss, a specific episode of confusion or a failure of someone to look after themselves may be a reason for someone to seek advice on behalf of an older person.

The third way that someone with memory problems can be detected by their GP is if there is a 'screening' procedure. Screening is a description of the system whereby tests are given to everybody who falls into a certain category (for example, over a certain age or in a particular practice) to try to detect a disease. Screening has somewhat fallen out of favour recently but still happens in some places.

The final way a memory problem can be brought to the attention of a GP is that a person may attend for something else (for example, a painful arm or a repeat prescription) and mention in passing that their memory has become poor. The process would then proceed as described on pages 93–4.

Memory clinics

These are specialist clinics which have grown up around the UK for the assessment (and sometimes treatment) of people with memory problems, including Alzheimer's disease and other dementias. They are multi-disciplinary (that is, they are run by different disciplines) but generally include a psychiatrist with a particular interest in older people and memory problems (an old age psychiatrist), nurses with a particular interest and experience in the area, and psychologists (who are not medically qualified but have specialist skills and expertise in the assessment and treatment of mental health problems). Other members of the team include occupational therapists (who are experts in maximizing a person's functional independence), speech and language therapists and social workers. As well as psychiatrists, specialists in general medicine in older people (geriatric medicine) can run memory clinics. These are doctors who have trained in hospital medicine but have chosen to specialize in the care of older people. Often, there is a close collaboration between colleagues in geriatric medicine and old age psychiatry.

At a memory clinic, the team will take a full history of the patient's memory problem and details about how it started and how it has progressed. Lots of other information about the patient and their history will also be taken.

Q **My doctor suggested that I get information about Alzheimer's disease from the Alzheimer's Society. Does this mean he doesn't know what he is talking about or doesn't care?**

A Absolutely not. The Alzheimer's Society is a phenomenal organization which supplies a great deal of up-to-date knowledge and advice on Alzheimer's disease as well as, in some areas, providing practical support. With no disrespect to doctors, the Society will know more about the practical aspects of care and where to access services and benefits. Your doctor is being particularly responsible and caring by suggesting you contact the Society.

Q My father was seen at the memory clinic and was diagnosed as having vascular dementia. He has a number of medical problems, including hypertension, raised cholesterol, and late onset diabetes. He was referred to a geriatrician (a physician specializing in the treatment of physical illness in older people). Does this mean there is something seriously wrong?

A No, it does not. Old age psychiatrists and geriatricians work very closely together, and some memory clinics are run by geriatricians. While an old age psychiatrist has a general knowledge of these medical conditions, he or she may feel that specialist advice is sometimes necessary.

The clinic will also carry out much more detailed examinations of memory and language function than is possible at a GP's surgery. The clinic may well arrange for tests including blood tests, one or more different types of brain scan and an electroencephalogram (EEG – a tracing of the brain waves). This process may take some time but then usually the patient would meet with a senior doctor who, with them and their family (or friends if they wish), will go through the results of all the tests and explain what the most likely cause of the problems is.

This could range from a diagnosis of Alzheimer's disease or vascular dementia (or a combination of the two) to another type of dementia. The tests may have uncovered a physical problem which needs attention by another specialist and the person would be referred on. It may be that the person has memory problems but that they do not amount to dementia. In this case, some help could be provided to improve their memory function and it is likely that they would be asked to go back to the clinic in a few months for another test of their memory to see if there has been any change. Their memory problems might be related to stress and they would have the opportunity to discuss this with the memory clinic staff. The person might have depression which would be treated in conjunction with their GP. A full report of the consultation would be sent to their GP and they are entitled to receive a copy, if they wish. If in doubt, they can ask for one.

Q **I have been referred to a memory clinic. Does that mean I have dementia?**

A Memory clinics are widespread and have been set up specifically to assess people complaining of memory problems. You must have some symptoms of memory loss for your doctor to seek a specialist opinion of the cause of that loss and to refer you to a memory clinic. It is quite common to have complaints of memory loss but no objective evidence of poor memory (where detailed tests of memory function are normal), in which case symptoms such as depression, anxiety and stress may be the cause and not dementia. So, referral to a memory clinic is an increasingly common and perfectly acceptable way to assess memory problems and you should not assume that because this has happened, you have dementia.

Old age psychiatry

There are around 450 specialists in the UK with a particular interest in **old age psychiatry**, that is a branch of psychiatry looking after older people (generally considered to be those over the age of 65). Old age psychiatrists deal with a whole range of mental health problems including dementia, depression and schizophrenia. They are generally based around the hospital and work within a multi-disciplinary team which includes nurses (specialist nurses who visit people in the community and community psychiatric nurses or CPNs), social workers, occupational therapists, physiotherapists and speech and language therapists. Old age psychiatrists tend to work both in hospitals and at home and see at lot of people in their own homes. Old age psychiatry teams, which are invariably linked to memory clinics, tend to care for people in the more advanced stages of dementia where a diagnosis has been made and perhaps established

old age psychiatry
This is a specialist discipline in medicine concerned with the treatment of mental disorders in older people (usually over the age of 65).

Q **What is a CPN?**

A This stands for Community Psychiatric Nurse. This person is a trained mental health nurse (many have a general nursing training as well) whose job is to support patients with mental health problems, and their families, in the community. This can take the form of supervision of medication, giving advice and practical help, and providing valuable support. They are based in specialist mental health teams, although more and more are attached to general practitioners. They are an invaluable source of support and help. Admiral Nurses are a relatively new development and are support workers primarily for the carers of people with dementia. They, too, work in the community.

for some years but people need supervision and extra advice and support in their own homes, in conjunction with other members of the multi-disciplinary team and Social Services.

Other medical disciplines

Neurologists are specialists in brain disease and deal with a whole range of neurological conditions including dementia, brain tumours, multiple sclerosis and epilepsy. Some have a particular interest and specialism in dementia. Neurologists tend to see people who are younger than those referred to old age psychiatrists but the range of tests and investigations are similar to those carried out in memory clinics. Geriatricians (specialists in the medicine of older people) sometimes have a particular interest in people with dementia but the majority of people they see are people with general medical conditions (for example, hypertension, diabetes, heart failure and strokes) who also have memory problems as part of that. As mentioned above, some geriatricians run memory clinics.

Although there are a number of specialists who can be involved in the assessment and diagnosis of dementia, the main continuing medical care and supervision is provided by the patient's GP.

Support at home

This support can take a number of different forms including regular visits by an old age psychiatrist, CPN and community team, and regular input from Social Services in terms of home helps, carers at home and social work visits. Support at home for patients and their carers is of the utmost importance. Maintaining a person's independence for as long as is possible and providing help for the carer is one of the cornerstones of effective management of dementia.

Drug treatment clinics

These are either part of a memory clinic and/or and old age psychiatry service, and in some areas in the UK they are a linked but related part of the service that deals specifically with the initiation and monitoring of drugs for Alzheimer's disease. The guidelines around the prescription of these drugs mean that detailed tests of memory and activities of daily living and other measures have to be made before the drugs are started and at regular intervals during their prescription. This is to ensure that the drugs are being used to their best effect. The assessments are coupled with the views of patients and carers as to whether the person has improved or not. In some ways the divisions between memory clinics, old age psychiatry services and drug treatment clinics are blurred but they are mentioned here because they do have separate functions and you may hear them being referred to in different ways. However, it is largely the same group of clinicians who look after each part of the service.

Nursing and residential care

When a person with dementia deteriorates and it is no longer practical for them to be cared for at home, consideration of admission to a nursing or residential home is often made. The distinction between nursing and residential care is becoming blurred but generally speaking, residential care is suitable for people who may have mild memory loss and need some supervision in managing themselves. They need more care than can be provided at home and more supervision than is given in sheltered accommodation. Nursing homes specialize in the physical care of older people who may have had a stroke or have severe heart failure or severe arthritis. There is a specialist type of home known by the outdated term 'ESMI' (which stands for Elderly Severely Mentally Infirm) which indicates people with quite severe dementia who usually have complex needs both in terms of physical care and behavioural problems that need specialist attention.

In some areas of the country there are specialist facilities in the community which deal with people with memory problems using new technologies, so-called 'smart' houses, where computer-driven aids can monitor an older person and maximize their ability to live independently. However, at present these are generally not available but should become much more common in the future. In some areas, continuing care for people suffering from very severe dementia is available on the NHS but generally only for people with very complex needs, such as people with persistent challenging behaviour which needs specialist clinical supervision and people with additional physical needs.

Every person is different and facilities vary from place to place but a typical course of somebody with early Alzheimer's disease is given below.

Living wills/advance directives

This is the situation when a person, while their memory and intellectual abilities are completely intact, makes a statement about how they would like to be cared for should they develop a condition such as dementia. They are just beginning to be more widely used in practice. It can be extremely helpful and reassuring for the clinical team looking after a person with Alzheimer's disease, and for their family, to be absolutely clear about the wishes of a person with dementia.

my experience

A journey through the care system

My mother was 76 when the family noticed that her memory was not quite as good as it had been. It was brought to our attention all of a sudden when she forgot the birthday of one of her grandchildren, generally regarded as a favourite whose birthday she had never forgotten before. When I met up with my brother and sisters they each had one or two examples over the previous two years of my mother's lapses of memory which, at the time, they tended to make a joke of and said it was just her age. My mother had been well all her life although recently had been bothered with some breathlessness and had arthritis in her hips but the pain was well controlled with anti-inflammatory drugs.

It took some months to persuade my mother to go with one of my sisters to the doctor. The doctor was newly qualified and had joined the practice recently and although she didn't know my mother, she had full access to all her notes. The doctor listened to what my sister said then asked my mother herself what she thought of her memory and then did a test there and then in the surgery by asking her to remember three words, then asking her to recall them after a couple of minutes, to recall a name and address that she had just made up and asked her questions about her general knowledge of things going on in the news.

After the examination, the GP arranged to see my mother again at the surgery to ask a few more questions and to get one of the practice nurses to take some blood. Following that, she said she was going to refer her to a memory clinic at the local hospital.

Within a month, the appointment arrived. When my mother went to the clinic she was seen by a nurse who went into great detail about her symptoms, how they had started, how they had progressed, all about her family history and what her expectation of the clinic was.

They arranged for some detailed tests of my mother's memory and arranged for a chest X-ray, CT brain scan and electroencephalogram. After about six weeks we got an appointment to see the consultant who was a woman, and who put my mother at ease straight away. She briefly went over the history again but did not go into a lot of detail as clearly that was already down in the notes. She then went through the results of all the tests – the blood tests from the GP and the results of the detailed tests of memory and all the various scans. She said that she thought that the most likely diagnosis was Alzheimer's disease. She talked about the various treatment options including prescribing one of the anti-dementia drugs and my mother seemed very keen to try this. I got the chance to ask questions about my mother's illness and, most importantly, what was likely to happen in the future.

My mother was still living alone at that time (she became a widow 12 years ago) but was managing fine with help from her family and from Social Services. The consultant asked for input from Social Services and within two weeks a Social Worker had visited my mother at home and suggested that she went to a day centre once a week. She started going there and enjoyed it greatly.

With regard to the drug treatment, she was seen by the consultant at another clinic and was started on one of the anti-dementia drugs. We noticed some improvements after about a month and the dose was increased. However, my mother then became sick and the dose was reduced. It was clear after about a year that she was not really any worse than she had been and everyone agreed that this was a success and she remained on the drug.

This situation went on for two or three years. There were odd moments of crisis – when she locked herself out one day and there was one day that everyone remembers during last summer when she went missing for about eight hours but was eventually found by the police and brought home (she had one of those identity bracelets on, thank goodness). Then suddenly, one day, I had a call from one of the care assistants who went in to look after my mother to say that she had found her unconscious. She had suffered a mild stroke and was admitted to hospital. She had some weakness down the left-hand side and her speech was slurred but with physiotherapy and speech therapy she regained about 90 per cent of her function. We had been increasingly concerned over the previous few months about her ability to manage at home despite input from Social Services. She was beginning to neglect her appearance, had lost weight and was not eating. She didn't look very well. We were all therefore quite relieved when the consultant in the general hospital said that he did not think my mother could go home and so we began looking for a residential home for her. My mother was adamant that she wanted to go home and we all told her how worried we were about her and finally she agreed to go into a home for a trial period.

We were very lucky to find one not far from where she lives and thankfully there was a bed available quite quickly. She settled in immediately and in fact made friends with someone she had known much earlier in her life but had not met for about 40 years.

Her dementia gradually increased and it became clear about three months after she had gone into the home that the anti-dementia drug was having no effect so we all agreed that it should be stopped. There was no change when it was stopped. We had heard on the radio about a new drug, memantine, which is available for people with more severe dementia but as my mother was so happy and content we did not think there was any reason to prescribe it and everyone agreed with us. She went into hospital a couple more times, once with an episode of heart failure which made her very confused and once with a urinary tract infection but she went back to the home without any problem.

She then became quite agitated and began shouting throughout the day and night. This was very difficult to control and very distressing for her, the staff and other residents. Eventually, a number of different drugs given in combination helped but she never really seemed to be the same after that. She stopped recognizing me and my brothers and sisters and in fact had not recognized her favourite grandson for a couple of years.

One day we got a phone call from the home to say that they had not been able to wake my mother up and her GP had seen her and diagnosed that she had had a major stroke. She never regained consciousness and died within 24 hours. The length of time from when she first saw her GP to when she died was six-and-a-half years.

CHAPTER

7

Caring for a person with dementia

The role of carers

It is very difficult to summarize in one chapter the many and varied roles that carers have in Alzheimer's disease. The topic is the subject of whole books in themselves and the reader is referred to a number of excellent sources of information regarding the pivotal role of carers. For example, the Alzheimer's Society devotes much of its time to providing advice to carers and its website (www.alzheimers.org.uk) is a mine of information. The classic text on the role of carers is *The 36 Hour Day* (Mace, N and Rabins, P, revised edition Warner Books, New York, 1992), the title emphasizing the terrible burden on carers. Another very useful book is *Alzheimer's Disease at your Fingertips* by Cayton, H, Graham, N and Warner, J (second edition, Class Publishing, London, 2002.)

While this book is primarily about Alzheimer's disease and its implications for the individual, it would be remiss not to include at least an overview of the role of carers. For convenience's sake, it is divided into the care of people with Alzheimer's disease in the early, moderate and more severe stages.

There is a large amount of research to show that caring for a patient with dementia is one of the most stressful things, and carers themselves pay a heavy price in terms of their own mental and physical health. For example, at any one time as many as two-thirds of carers suffer from depression and there is good evidence to suggest that their own physical health suffers as well. It is the abnormal behaviours and psychiatric symptoms (the so-called neuropsychiatric features) which cause most strain and this is totally understandable. In the early stages, subtle changes in mood, emotions and personality occur and these symptoms tend to be more severe as the disease progresses.

It has been said that the things which put most strain on carers of people with Alzheimer's disease are those things that parents find most troublesome in children – for example, constant questioning, being up a great deal at night, incontinence (bedwetting in children) and following a person around constantly (known as trailing).

Early stages

It may be that in the early stages the sufferer does not notice the first signs of memory loss, although often in retrospect they will appreciate that they had perhaps lost their keys, forgotten an important event, such as a birthday, or had begun to forget people's names. Along with this,

myth
Memory loss is always the first sign of Alzheimer's disease.

fact
No, subtle changes in personality and changes in emotional reaction can often be the first sign that something is going wrong. However, it can be quite hard to separate these changes from normal ageing and it is usually only in retrospect that one can recognize that something has changed.

subtle emotional changes, such as irritability, occur and, again in retrospect, carers often describe how subtle changes in personality and a hardening of the emotions (the so-called coarsening effect) may occur. These changes are often put down to the normal effects of ageing and, in many cases, that will be the case but in a proportion, they represent the initial stages of the dementia.

Generally, in Alzheimer's disease, it is long-term memory (in this context, memory for events going back 20 or 30 years) that is relatively preserved, whereas short-term memory (a few minutes) is lost. This can cause some consternation in relatives who do not appreciate that memory can vary like this and it can be frustrating as the carer may think that the person is doing something on purpose. An approach which is beginning to become more common is called 'post-diagnostic counselling'. This is a specific programme of advice and education instigated after a diagnosis has been made, usually at an out-patient clinic. It can provide a great deal of help and support to carers.

The most important aspect of understanding the role and the attitudes of carers in Alzheimer's disease is that a carer's reaction cannot be seen in isolation and is usually a result not just of their own personality but the relationship which they have had with the patient, often over many, many years. Irritations, frictions and annoyances can become magnified and the carer's reaction exaggerated. To scold someone with early Alzheimer's disease who has lost their keys seems inappropriate but if the person refuses, for example, to put their keys in the same place all the time as an aid to remembering where they are, it is more understandable that it will attract negative comment.

In the early stages, particularly, patients will try to hide and cover up these lapses and this can create tension. A patient may accuse a carer of forgetting to remind them of a particular event and this can cause friction. Although it is easier to say than do, it can be a salutary lesson for a carer to imagine themselves in the place of a patient with failing faculties to see how they themselves might react. The way that we view the world is called our **attributional style**. Some people have a negative attributional style in that they have a tendency to blame others for what happens. An example in Alzheimer's disease would be a man who becomes aggressive. If his wife or child is of the opinion that it is his illness that is causing him to have a change of character and be aggressive, then it is easy to manage and understand. Compare this to the situation where a carer may think that the person is being aggressive on purpose. This situation might bring back unhappy memories of aggression earlier on.

Often, a carer's reaction to a certain behaviour tells one more about the carer themselves and their relationship to the patient rather than anything specific about the behaviour. This is often seen when two patients may have a similar degree of behavioural disturbance while the carers react very differently, perhaps one being more understanding and forgiving and one having a very low tolerance threshold for anything that goes wrong. One can often be surprised at how long some relatives can care for a person at home whereas others have a much lower

attributional style
A person's way of interpreting things around them.

threshold, demanding admission to a nursing or residential home.

Moderate stages

At this stage, neuropsychiatric features begin to emerge and there are some specific symptoms which deserve special mention.

One of the most distressing symptoms is where a patient fails to recognize their carer and this is much more than simply forgetting someone's name. It seems to relate to specific areas of damage in the brain which control the process of recognition. In an extreme form, a person may even imagine that a loved one has been replaced by someone else (an imposter) and this can cause particular stress. An unusual feature which impinges on carers is where there is misidentification with reduplication – the most common being when a person with Alzheimer's disease feels they have two houses and spends time worrying about getting back to the other house rather than the strange one in which they invariably find themselves. A practical way of managing this is simply to take the patient out on a short journey in the car or bus, or on a walk and then return to the same house. Not infrequently, the patient will be relieved that they have returned safely.

A question which is regularly asked is how much should a carer 'go along' with an abnormal belief and how much should they challenge it. There is no right or wrong answer to this and probably the best advice is to tread a middle ground. For example, if a patient begins to say that their wife is not really their wife but a stranger, then it is appropriate and a natural human response to try to gently indicate to the patient that they are incorrect. However, going to exhaustive lengths by constantly looking through old photograph albums and even getting a marriage certificate to prove the person is wrong, is not helpful and is liable to cause more distress and trouble. Remember that the person truly believes what they think – they are not making it up and no one enjoys being proved wrong, especially when they believe they are right. In a similar way, if a person is disoriented to time and place, a gentle reminder of the correct time and the correct situation is entirely appropriate but then one should leave it at that and not take it any further. A common mistake which doctors tend to make is when an elderly person in their eighties claims that their parents are alive and living at home; the doctor tries to get the patient to calculate what age their parents would be to try and reorientate them but the logic of the argument is invariably lost and often causes more distress. (One has to be aware as well, that someone in their eighties could well have parents who are alive and over 100!)

In the moderate stages, there is often the beginnings of difficulties in activities of daily living, such as an inability to dress correctly and the person may need help in choosing clothes. It may be that the carer has to lower their expectations in terms of sartorial style and perhaps lower previously held standards. For example, if it takes a person an hour to get ready, rather than getting angry and frustrated at possibly being late for something, just start an hour earlier. If a person insists on wearing a shirt for perhaps two or three days, is that the end of the world? There is a thin line to tread between lowering expectations to

Q **My wife thinks her parents are still alive when in reality they died over 30 years ago. Should I correct her?**

A It depends if it causes her or you any distress. If it is just a casual belief she mentions from time to time and it does no harm, then it is probably best to ignore it. However, if she is constantly searching for her parents and is clearly distressed when she cannot find them, some gentle reinforcing of the fact that they are dead could be helpful. However, remember that because she has no recollection of the death, she may have a bereavement reaction and may experience the loss very acutely each time she is told.

Q **My husband has Alzheimer's disease and is aggressive and sometimes pushes me. Should I push him back?**

A You obviously need to feel safe with your husband and it is unacceptable to live in fear of what he might do. However, remember that it is his illness that is making him react the way he does and simply to retaliate will achieve nothing and will inevitably make matters worse. It may be that you could begin to develop strategies to remove yourself from the situation if you are able to anticipate when he will become aggressive, although ultimately it may be that some medication may be needed.

accommodate the deficits that occur with the disease and maintaining a good standard of function and living. Remember, as the carer, you are invariably the person who knows the sufferer best and you are in the best position to make judgements about what is right for the patient. Make sure it is right for them, though, and not for yourself.

Severe stages

In the most severe stages, there can often be very practical issues with regard to dressing, eating and going to the toilet as well as the emergence of some distressing behaviours such as aggression, agitation, paranoid beliefs and sexual disinhibitions. Again, there is no blanket way of reacting to and managing these distressing symptoms but sometimes it can be helpful to stand back and do what is called an 'ABC analysis'. This consists of looking at the Antecedents (events that led up to a particular behaviour), the Behaviours themselves and analysis of the Consequences of the behaviour.

For example, an elderly woman with Alzheimer's disease becomes agitated and paces around in the late afternoon and early evening. It can be helpful to recognize the consistency of the time (Antecedent) of the Behaviour (to plan interventions) because the behaviour itself may be due to the woman going back in time and imagining that she has to get her husband's tea ready when he comes in from work, and the Consequence is that a person may stand at a particular door for an hour or two in an evening.

An understanding of the possible reasons behind the behaviour and its exact consequences is the first stage to understanding it more and being able to plan a strategy to manage it. For example, if that situation occurs in a nursing or residential home, then the staff should be aware that this behaviour happens most evenings (Antecedent) and so it should not come as a surprise when it does happen. The Behaviour itself is understandable in terms of what the person is doing, and perhaps engaging them in conversation about their husband might help. One also has to decide whether the Consequence of the behaviour, that is a person hanging around a particular door, is a cause of great concern or not. It may be that directing the person towards the kitchen, perhaps to help with laying the tables, might do a lot to make the behaviour less obvious.

It is hard to do justice to the wide array of complex changes which occur in a person with Alzheimer's disease and the way they should be best managed. The reader is strongly advised to seek out other sources of information and in particular to address any specific concerns that you may have.

myth
Drugs are the best way of managing abnormal behaviours.

fact
Many drugs have side effects and a great deal of good can be done by using non-drug approaches to the management of behaviours such as understanding the causes and the meaning of them.

my experience

My husband was diagnosed as having Alzheimer's disease when he was 72. The first time I noticed something was wrong when he forgot our wedding anniversary, which he had never done before. He became increasingly confused after that and used to be very irritable with me. One day he said that I was not his wife and that I had been replaced by an imposter. I was very frightened and I thought he had gone mad. He seemed very calm and said that he was very happy living with me although he knew I was not his wife. On a couple of occasions he thought that there was someone else in the house and I began to turn the mirrors round as he used to catch his reflection, not recognize himself and then accuse me of having an affair with the man he saw in the mirror. When we were much younger we had some marital problems and I did in fact have a brief affair but only for six months and then it ended. I am sure he never knew about it but it upset me greatly that he said this and I felt incredibly guilty.

Things went from bad to worse and he got a urinary tract infection and was admitted to hospital where he was very confused and hit the staff a number of times and he was given drugs to sedate him. He came home but within a few days had to be re-admitted because he became aggressive again. He had a stroke, sadly, and died a few days later.

CHAPTER

8 Ten ways to improve your memory

1 DON'T PANIC! Allow yourself the time to remember the information, it doesn't matter if this takes a little longer.

2 Try to imagine where you were when you first heard or saw the information that you are trying to recall. Put yourself back in the same context as vividly as possible.

3 Pen and paper are the most useful tools to aid your memory. If your memory is not very good, write things down. Do this for even fairly mundane things because when someone asks you what you did yesterday, you can come up with an answer, rather than, 'I can't remember', which is not helpful for your confidence. Attach a pen or pencil to the notepad and keep it with you as much as you can. Having post-it notes can be extremely helpful as well. Some people carry a card with important numbers on them but beware that banks say we should never write down our PIN numbers for our bank accounts. Diaries work well because they can help you to organize information and also keep you in touch with days and dates.

4 Try to 'muster up' all your concentration when carrying out an activity or taking in information that you may be liable to forget. Try to repeat the information back to yourself from time to time, for example, 'Her name is Catherine'.

5 Combine a visual image with words, for example, 'Her name is Catherine and she has curly hair'.

6 Keep everything in its place as far as is possible. For example, keys and spectacles are easy to misplace, so put them down in the same place whenever you can. Again, when you put them down try to 'visualize' the place in order to jog your memory. If you put your keys on to a specific table, imagine the table carved into the shape of a giant key. The more humorous and larger than life the image, the more likely you are to remember it.

7 If you need to take a certain object with you when going out, for example, an umbrella, put it in front of the door, perhaps on the mat. You will have to step over it to go out and you will see it and remember it.

8 Use 'stick it' notes in prominent places. For example, near the cooker or on the back of the kitchen door – 'SWITCH OFF COOKER', 'PUT LIGHTS OUT'. Also, cupboards can be labelled with the names of the objects that go inside.

9 Go through the alphabet if you need to in order to remember a name or word.

10 Be honest! 'My memory is not as good as it used to be' will often take the pressure off you, and many people can relate to this. Everyone recognizes that you have to adapt your life if you have a sore back, a hip replacement or diabetes, and it is just the same with having a poor memory. Most older people will experience some decline in their memory, and almost everyone will have had instances during their lifetime when their memory has been less than perfect.

Further help

Useful addresses

Age Concern England
Astral House
1268 London Road
London SW16 4ER
Tel: 020 8765 7200
Email: ace@ace.org.uk
Web: www.ace.org.uk

Age Concern Scotland
Leonard Small House
113 Rose Street
Edinburgh EH2 3DT
Tel: 0131 220 3345
Email: enquiries@acscot.org.uk
Web: www.ageconcernscotland.
org. uk

Alzheimer's Scotland
22 Drumsheugh Gardens
Edinburgh EH3 7RN
Tel: 0131 243 1453
Email: alzheimer@alzscot.org
Web: www.alzscot.org

Alzheimer's Society
Gordon House
10 Greencoat Place
London SW1P 1PH
Tel: 020 7306 0606
Email: enquiries@alzheimers.org.uk
Web: www.alzheimers.org.uk

Carers National Association
20/25 Glasshouse Yard
London EC1A 4JT
Tel: 020 7490 8818
Carers Line: 0345 573 369
Web: www.londonhealth.co.uk/
carersnationalassociation.asp

CJD Support Network
Po Box 346
Market Drayton
Shropshire
TF9 4WN
Helpline: 01630 673973
Tel: 01630 673993
Email: Info@cjdsupport.net
Web: www.cjdsupport.net

Crossroads Association
10 Regent Place
Rugby
Warwickshire CV21 2PN
Tel: 0845 450 0350
Email: communications@
crossroads.org.uk
Web: www.crossroads.org.uk

**National Creutzfeldt-Jakob
Disease
Surveillance Unit**
Western General Hospital
Crewe Road
Edinburgh EH4 2XU
Tel: 0131 537 2128
Web: www.cjd.ed.ac.uk

Parkinson's Disease Society
215 Vauxhall Bridge Road
London SW1V 1EJ
Tel: 020 7931 8080
Email: enquiries@parkinsons.org.uk
Web: www.parkinsons.org.uk

Picks Disease Support Group
Advisor, 8 Brooksby Close
Oadby
Leicester
LE2 5AB
Tel: 0845 458 3208
Email: carol@pdsg.org.uk
Web: www.pdsg.org.uk/organisers

Public Guardianship Office
Archway Tower
2 Junction Road
London N19 5SZ
Tel: 0845 330 2900
Email: custserv@
guardianship.gov.uk
Web: www.guardianship.gov.uk

Helpful websites

Age Exchange
www.age-exchange.org.uk
Age Exchange co-ordinates the European Reminiscence Network which teaches family carers and volunteers reminiscence skills and activities as a way of using the long-term memory of people with dementia to enhance communication and lessen social isolation.

Alzheimer's Society
www.alzheimers.org.uk
The leading UK care and research charity for people with dementia, their families and carers.

Better Caring
www.bettercaring.co.uk
A website that will help you to find care homes and also proclaims to 'answer all your care questions'.

Carers UK
www.carersuk.org
A site for anyone providing care for a relative or friend. Run by carers who campaign for a better deal for carers and provide information to support them.

Counsel and care
www.counselandcare.org.uk
Help and advice for anyone over 60.

for dementia
www.fordementia.org.uk
This website promotes and develops admiral nursing – a specialist nursing intervention focused on meeting the needs of carers and supporters of people with dementia; it also offers training for carers.

Memoryclinic.com
www.memoryclinic.com
Gives information about memory loss and its treatment along with news and an 'ask the expert' facility. Includes the National Memory Test which users can complete (fee currently £1.50). Some pages can be viewed only after initial registration (this is free).

Glossary

activities of daily living
Things which we carry out in our everyday lives and which are affected in someone suffering from dementia. Examples include dressing, feeding, washing, eating, handling money, shopping, driving and using the telephone.

Alzheimer's disease
The most common cause of dementia affecting about 60 per cent of people with dementia.

anticholinesterase drugs
A new type of drug which improves the symptoms of Alzheimer's disease by raising the level of a neurotransmitter, acetylcholine, in the brain.

'apparent phase' of dementia
Where people other than the sufferer become aware of the disease.

arthrosclerotic plaque
A general term indicating the presence of the deposition of something abnormal – senile plaques can be seen deposited in the brain in between nerve fibres in Alzheimer's disease. Deposits of fat in arteries occur as part of normal ageing process and predipose strokes, heart attacks and vascular dementia.

attributional style A person's way of interpreting things around them.

autosomal dominant condition A condition passed from generation to generation even if only one parent is affected. (An autosomal recessive condition needs both parents to be affected for it to be passed on.)

behavioural disturbances Behaviours such as wandering, agitation, aggression and sexual disinhibition seen in people with dementia.

cerebrospinal fluid Cerebrospinal fluid is the fluid which bathes the brain – it is inside the brain substance and also around the outside of the brain. It is a way of cushioning the brain from forces from outside. The fluid is manufactured inside the brain and circulates to the outside (still inside the skull) where it is absorbed into the bloodstream. If there is any blockage to that circulation, the amount of fluid under pressure can build up, giving hydrocephalus. In children, before the skull bones have knitted together, this causes an increase in the size of the head but after about 18 months or 2 years of age, the skull is firm and the pressure, as it increases inside, squashes the brain rather than causing the head to enlarge.

cerebrovascular disease Any disease affecting an artery within the brain, or supplying blood to the brain.

cognitive function Tests of memory, language and mental agility carried out to test the brain's function.

confusion A commonly used term indicating, usually, that a person does not know where they are and/or does not know the date, and/or does things which are inappropriate.

court of protection An official part of the court system which protects a person who, through dementia or any other mental illness, has lost the ability to handle their affairs.

CT (computed tomography) scan A type of brain scan which shows the structure of the brain.

delirium The acute upset in mental function causing disorientation, confusion and psychiatric symptoms such as auditory and visual hallucination and paranoid ideas. It tends to come on quickly as it is invariably caused by physical illness.

delusions False ideas which are fixed and unshakeable and often seen in people with dementia.

dementia A condition of the brain, with a number of causes, which gives rise to memory loss and emotional changes and results in a person having difficulty looking after themselves.

depression A state of lowered mood seen commonly in people with dementia.

differential diagnosis The range of possible conditions that can mimic the symptoms of dementia.

Down's syndrome Down's syndrome refers to a congenital disorder where a characteristically flattened facial appearance, short stature and low IQ is present. It is caused by an individual having 3 copies (instead of the normal 2) of chromosome 21. It used to be called Mongolism but this term was regarded as offensive and is now no longer used.

electrocardiogram (ECG) A tracing of the heart showing the rate (number of beats per minute) as well as showing if the electrical conduction of the heart is normal. It can also be used to diagnose heart attacks.

electroencephalogram (EEG) A tracing of the brain waves which can be used to diagnose epilepsy. It can also show where there is shrinkage of the brain and is used to diagnose Creutzfeldt–Jakob disease.

errorless learning A technique that prevents errors from being made during training.

frontal lobe dementia	A type of dementia caused by shrinkage in the front part of the brain.
GP	General practitioner (doctor).
hallucinations	Experiences such as visual or auditory hallucinations (seeing or hearing things when there is nothing there) seen in people with dementia.
'hidden phase' of dementia	A very mild and subtle change in memory which may not be regarded as abnormal.
hydrocephalus	This refers to an increased amount of the normal fluid (cerebrospinal fluid) which lies around the brain, inside the skull.
Lewy body dementia	A type of dementia caused by deposits of protein called Lewy bodies.
memory clinic	An out-patient clinic specializing in the diagnosis and treatment of people with memory disorders.
misidentifications	When a person with dementia does not recognize a person or an object.
MRI (magnetic resource imaging) scan	A type of brain scan which shows the structure of the brain in finer detail compared to a CT scan.
neuropsychiatric symptoms	A number of psychiatric or psychological symptoms and behavioural disturbances seen in dementia.
neuropsychological features	Part of the expression of dementia characterized by amnesia (loss of memory), aphasia (problems understanding or expressing words), agnosia (failure to recognize people or objects) and apraxia (the inability to carry out tasks such as writing, dressing or using a knife and fork).
neurotransmitter	A chemical messenger in the brain which allows messages to be sent between brain cells (neurons).

old age psychiatry	This is a specialist discipline in medicine concerned with the treatment of mental disorders in older people (usually over the age of 65).
psychiatric symptoms	Symptoms such as depression, delusions, hallucinations and misidentification seen in people with dementia.
psychotic symptoms	Symptoms such as delusions, hallucinations and misidentifications.
reduplication	When a person suffering from Alzheimer's disease thinks that there are two of something – an object or a person – usually something which has emotional significance to the sufferer.
spaced retrieval technique	A teaching method that involves the recall of information at short intervals initially, with a gradual increase in the time span.
SPET scan (Single Photon Emission Tomography)	A type of brain scan that shows the blood flow in the brain.
vanishing cues	The attempts to improve verbal memory skills by giving letters/numbers as clues to a required answer.
vascular dementia	The second most common cause of dementia affecting about 20 per cent of people with dementia.

# Sources of figures and plates

Figure 1
CT scan machine. Science Photo Library/AJ Photo/Hop American
Figure 2
MRI scan machine. Science Photo Library/John Cole
Figure 3
Visual imagery

Plate 1
A CT scan of a normal brain. Courtesy of the Department of Medical Illustration, Withington Hospital, Manchester.
Plate 2
A CT scan showing shrinkage of the brain (atrophy) in Alzheimer's disease. Courtesy of the Department of Medical Illustration, Withington Hospital, Manchester.
Plate 3
A CT scan showing shrinkage of the front part of the brain. Courtesy of the Department of Medical Illustration, Withington Hospital, Manchester.
Plate 4
A CT scan showing a brain tumour. Courtesy of the Department of Medical Illustration, Withington Hospital, Manchester.

Plate 5

A CT scan showing normal pressure hydrocephalus. Courtesy of the Department of Medical Illustration, Withington Hospital, Manchester.

Plate 6

A CT scan showing an area where the brain has died as a result of a cerebral infarction (stroke). Courtesy of the Department of Medical Illustration, Withington Hospital, Manchester.

Plate 7

An MRI scan showing a normal brain. Courtesy of Professor John O'Brien, University of Newcastle.

Plate 8

An MRI scan showing atrophy in Alzheimer's disease. Courtesy of Professor John O'Brien, University of Newcastle.

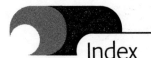

Index

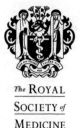

The ROYAL
SOCIETY of
MEDICINE

The Royal Society of Medicine (RSM) is an independent medical charity with a primary aim to provide continuing professional development for qualified medical and health-related professionals. The public benefits from health care professionals who have received high quality and relevant education from the RSM.

The Society celebrated its bicentenary in 2005. Each year it arranges and holds over 400 meetings for health care professionals across a wide range of medical subjects. In order to aid education and training further the Society also has the largest postgraduate medical library in Europe – based in central London together with online access to specialist databases. RSM Press, the Society's publishing arm, publishes books and journals principally aimed at the medical profession.

A number of conferences and events are held each year for the public as well as members of the Society. These include the successful 'Medicine and me' series, designed to bring together patients, their carers and the medical profession. In addition the RSM's Open and History of Medicine Sections arrange meetings on a regular basis which can be attended by the public.

In addition to the lectures and training provided by the RSM, members of the Society also have access to club facilities including accommodation and a restaurant. The conference and meeting facilities of the RSM were refurbished for their bicentenary and are available to the public for hire for meetings and seminars. In addition, Chandos House, a beautifully restored Georgian townhouse, designed by Robert Adam, is also now available to hire for training, receptions and weddings (as it has a civil wedding licence).

To find out more about the Royal Society of Medicine and the work it undertakes please visit www.rsm.ac.uk or call 020 7290 2991. For more information about RSM Press, please visit www.rsmpress.co.uk.